Quantum Healing

Healing and Being Through Mastering Energy

(Quantum Healing Meditation Techniques to Rewire Your Mind in Minutes)

Thomas Ellington

Published By **Jenna Olsen**

Thomas Ellington

Quantum Healing: Healing and Being Through Mastering Energy (Quantum Healing Meditation Techniques to Rewire Your Mind in Minutes)

ISBN 978-0-9958610-5-3

Legal & Disclaimer

The information contained in this book is not designed to replace or take the place of any form of medicine or professional medical advice. The information in this book has been provided for educational & entertainment purposes only.

The information contained in this book has been compiled from sources deemed reliable, and it is accurate to the best of the Author's knowledge; however, the Author cannot guarantee its accuracy and validity and cannot be held liable for any errors or omissions. Changes are periodically made to this book. You must consult your doctor or get professional medical advice before using any of the suggested remedies, techniques, or information in this book.

Upon using the information contained in this book, you agree to hold harmless the Author from and against any damages, costs, and expenses, including any legal fees potentially resulting from the application of any of the information provided by this guide. This disclaimer applies to any damages or injury caused by the use and application, whether directly or indirectly, of any advice or information presented, whether for breach of contract, tort, negligence, personal injury, criminal intent, or under any other cause of action.

You agree to accept all risks of using the information presented inside this book. You need to consult a professional medical practitioner in order to ensure you are both able and healthy enough to participate in this program.

Table Of Contents

Chapter 1: Exploring The Concept Of Quantum Wellness

In extremely-modern fast-paced global, wherein pressure and anxiety have come to be a vital a part of our lives, the idea of quantum properly being has emerged as a beacon of desire. But what exactly does it imply? Quantum well being is a holistic method to well-being that encompasses the thoughts, frame, and spirit, focusing on the interconnectedness of all factors of our being. It delves into the sector of quantum physics, wherein strength and consciousness intertwine, offering a ultra-modern attitude on fitness and healing.

At its center, quantum properly being acknowledges that we are not just bodily beings but furthermore active beings. It recognizes that our thoughts, emotions, and ideals have a profound impact on our usual nicely-being. Quantum physics teaches us that the entirety within the universe is made from electricity, which includes our bodies and minds. By records and harnessing this power, we will tap into our innate recovery abilities and achieve maximum useful properly being.

Quantum properly being emphasizes the power of cause and mindfulness. It encourages us to come to be aware of our mind and emotions, as they immediately have an effect on our energy place. By cultivating terrific mind and emotions, we will increase our vibration frequency, attracting greater best opinions into our lives. This idea aligns with the regulation of appeal, which states that like draws like. By that specialize in what we want in desire to what we do no longer need, we can take region our dreams and create a lifestyles of abundance and properly-being.

Furthermore, quantum well being recognizes the interconnectedness of all residing beings. It acknowledges that we aren't damage loose our environment however alternatively deeply linked to it. Just as our thoughts and feelings have an effect on our energy subject, furthermore they have got an impact on the world round us. By cultivating love, compassion, and gratitude, we're able to radiate extraordinary electricity, developing a ripple effect that extends beyond ourselves. This interconnectedness extends to our relationships as nicely. By nurturing healthy and harmonious connections with others, we're able to enhance our not unusual nicely-being.

Quantum well-being additionally embraces opportunity recovery modalities that artwork with the body's energy subject. Practices including acupuncture, Reiki, and power recuperation aim to repair stability and concord within the body, selling restoration on a physical, emotional, and non secular diploma. These modalities recognize that contamination and ailment are frequently a cease stop result of imbalances in our power difficulty and are trying to find to cope with the muse cause rather than definitely the symptoms.

In essence, quantum well being invites us to take an lively characteristic in our personal recovery journey. It encourages us to find out our ideals, release limiting styles, and embody a more holistic method to nicely-being. By integrating the thoughts of quantum physics into our lives, we are able to faucet into the limitless capability inside us and create a existence of colorful fitness, pride, and fulfillment.

In conclusion, the idea of quantum health offers a easy mindset on fitness and restoration It invitations us to explore the interconnectedness of our thoughts, frame, and spirit, and harness the power of our thoughts and emotions. By embracing this holistic technique, we are able to tap into our innate healing abilities and create lifestyles of most reliable well-being. So, permit us to embark on this adventure of self-discovery and unfastened up the infinite potential inner us, as we discover the fascinating global of quantum wellness.

The Connection between Mind and Body in Quantum Wellness: Unveiling the Intricacies of Holistic Harmony

In the world of wellness, a profound and fascinating phenomenon emerges whilst we discover the complex connection maximum of the thoughts and frame. Quantum well-being, a idea rooted in the ideas of quantum physics, delves into the profound interplay amongst our thoughts, feelings, and physical properly-being. This captivating exploration unveils a world wherein the mind and frame are not separate entities however instead interconnected components of our being, influencing every extraordinary in methods that move beyond traditional knowledge.

At the coronary heart of quantum properly-being lies the belief that our thoughts and emotions very own a vibration frequency that may affect our bodily fitness. Quantum physics teaches us that everything inside the universe, alongside facet our mind and emotions, includes strength. This strength, even as harnessed and directed consciously, can create a harmonious stability between the mind and frame, leading to stepped forward properly-being and electricity.

The thoughts, frequently considered the epicenter of our recognition, holds great strength over our bodily state. Our mind and ideals shape our fact, influencing the manner we understand and revel in the sector round us. Quantum nicely being acknowledges that horrible thoughts and emotions can manifest as physical illnesses, at the equal time as great thoughts and feelings can sell recuperation and everyday fitness.

The mind-frame connection in quantum health is not limited to the arena of thoughts and feelings on my own. It extends to the very material of our being, encompassing our cell shape and the energy that flows internal us. Quantum nicely-being recognizes that our bodies aren't merely bodily vessels however as an opportunity complicated systems of energy, continuously interacting with the quantum area that permeates the universe.

When we align our thoughts, feelings, and intentions with the quantum subject, we faucet proper into a limitless deliver of healing and transformation This alignment allows us to get right of access to the innate information of our bodies, permitting us to heal from inside and restore stability on all ranges. Quantum nicely-being empowers us to grow to be energetic members in our very own well-being, recognizing that we own the functionality to influence our fitness through aware reason and focused energy.

The practice of quantum well being encompasses severa modalities that facilitate the mind-body connection. Meditation, for example, serves as a effective device to quiet the mind, permitting us to faucet into our internal knowledge and connect to the quantum discipline. Through meditation, we're capable of domesticate a kingdom of deep rest and heightened recognition, fostering a harmonious courting among our mind, feelings, and physical body.

Another essential aspect of quantum fitness is the electricity of visualization. By vividly imagining our favored state of properly-being, we're able to harness the quantum discipline to expose up our intentions into fact. Visualization strategies allow us to create a intellectual blueprint of our best health, activating the thoughts-frame connection and beginning a cascade of superb modifications inner our being.

Furthermore, quantum nicely-being acknowledges the importance of energy recovery practices which incorporates Reiki, acupuncture, and sound remedy these modalities paintings at the precept that energy imbalances inside the body can result in bodily and emotional disharmony. By channeling healing energy into unique factors or areas of the frame, those practices repair stability and sell holistic fitness.

In the arena of quantum fitness, the mind and body aren't separate entities however as an possibility interconnected additives of our being. By acknowledging and nurturing this connection, we release the functionality for profound healing and transformation. Quantum nicely-being invites us to find out the depths of our popularity, harness the power of our thoughts and feelings, and include the countless opportunities that lie interior us.

In stop, the relationship among the thoughts and frame in quantum health is a charming and transformative journey. It unveils the difficult interplay among our thoughts, emotions, and physical nicely-being, highlighting the profound impact our reputation has on our health. By embracing the necessities of quantum physics and aligning our mind, feelings, and intentions with the quantum subject, we are able to faucet right right into a countless supply of restoration and nicely-being. Quantum properly-being empowers us to come to be energetic individuals in our personal health, fostering a harmonious dating between the mind and body, and unlocking the functionality for holistic harmony.

Understanding the Principles of Holistic Healing in Quantum Wellness

Holistic healing is a concept that has received large recognition in contemporary years, as human beings are more and more seeking out possibility strategies to their health and well-being. One such approach is quantum fitness, which combines the thoughts of quantum physics with holistic healing practices. By expertise the thoughts of holistic healing in quantum properly-being, people can tap into the energy in their mind, body, and spirit to gain most dependable fitness and nicely-being.

At its center, holistic recuperation acknowledges that the mind, body, and spirit are interconnected and that genuine recovery can handiest upward thrust up whilst all factors of someone are in stability. Quantum wellbeing takes this idea a step in addition through manner of incorporating the concepts of quantum physics, which suggest that the entirety in the universe is crafted from electricity and that this electricity is interconnected.

One of the critical element standards of quantum properly-being is the concept that our mind and emotions have an immediate effect on our physical health. Quantum physics teaches us that our thoughts and emotions emit vibrations or frequencies that may every sell fitness or make a contribution to contamination. By expertise this principle, humans can learn how to harness the energy of their thoughts and emotions to promote recuperation and well-being.

Another principle of quantum nicely being is the concept of energy recuperation. Quantum physics suggests that the whole lot within the universe is fabricated from strength, which embody our our bodies. When our strength will become imbalanced or blocked, it can bring about physical, emotional, and non secular illnesses. Energy healing practices, which includes Reiki or acupuncture, artwork to repair the go with the flow of strength within the frame, selling recovery and nicely-being.

In addition to power restoration, quantum wellness moreover consists of the usage of vibrational remedy. Vibrational remedy is based totally mostly on the principle that top notch frequencies of energy could have a profound impact on our fitness and nicely-being. This can consist of using sound remedy, shade therapy, or maybe the use of precise frequencies to promote recuperation.

Chapter 2: The Role Of Energy In Mind-Body Healing

In contemporary years, there was a developing hobby in exploring the characteristic of energy in mind-frame restoration. This growing place of have a take a look at suggests that energy, at a quantum degree, performs a essential position within the favored nicely-being and healing of an man or woman. By information and harnessing this power, we may additionally moreover free up new opportunities for healing and transformation.

To comprehend the region of strength in thoughts-frame restoration, we want to first delve into the sector of quantum physics. Quantum physics is a branch of technological know-how that explores the behavior of remember huge range and energy on the smallest scales. It well-known a worldwide this is an prolonged way from the deterministic and predictable nature of classical physics. Instead, it introduces us to a realm of uncertainty, interconnectedness, and limitless opportunities.

At the coronary coronary heart of quantum physics lies the idea of energy. Energy isn't merely a bodily strain; it is the essence of everything that exists. It is the underlying cloth of the universe, connecting all depend and cognizance. In this angle, the mind and frame aren't separate entities but as a substitute interconnected factors of a unified entire.

When we preserve in mind the position of energy in mind-frame restoration, we need to renowned that our our our our bodies aren't simply bodily entities. They are also composed of diffused energy fields that have interaction with the bigger energetic matrix of the universe. These power fields, often known as the biofield or air of thriller, are believed to be responsible for retaining our trendy fitness and nicely-being.

From a quantum attitude, contamination and illness aren't completely physical manifestations but as an alternative imbalances or disruptions in the electricity go with the glide inside our bodies. When the energy go together with the waft is blocked or stagnant, it is able to reason physical, emotional, and intellectual imbalances. By addressing those lively imbalances, we can restore concord and facilitate the restoration device.

One of the maximum captivating factors of energy recuperation is the idea of aim. Intention is the conscious direction of power toward a selected final effects. It is the targeted interest and perception that our mind and emotions have the energy to steer our bodily reality. Quantum physics shows that our intentions can right away effect the active area round us, affecting our health and well-being.

Numerous strength restoration modalities have emerged that harness the power of intention and strength to promote thoughts-body recovery. Reiki, for example, is a

Japanese approach that consists of the switch of strength thru the practitioner's hands to the recipient. This power waft facilitates to take away lively blockages, restore stability, and promote restoration on all levels.

Another modality gaining reputation is acupuncture, an ancient Chinese exercise that entails the insertion of skinny needles into unique elements at the frame. According to conventional Chinese treatment, those factors correspond to energy meridians that modify the go along with the drift of Qi, or existence stress strength. By stimulating those factors, acupuncture targets to restore the stability of energy and promote restoration.

Sound healing is however some other modality that makes use of electricity to facilitate thoughts-frame healing. Sound has been used for masses of years as a powerful device for recovery and transformation. Through the usage of particular frequencies and vibrations, sound recuperation objectives to harmonize the active place, launch stagnant electricity, and promote ordinary well-being.

While the concept of strength recovery can also moreover seem esoteric or mystical to some, it's miles essential to be conscious that medical research is starting to validate its efficacy. Studies have proven that strength recuperation modalities which includes Reiki and acupuncture can also need to have big first-rate effects on ache manipulate, pressure bargain, and regular well-being. These findings offer a scientific basis for the placement of power in mind-body recovery.

In cease, the position of power in thoughts-body healing is a fascinating and promising issue of examine. By knowledge and harnessing the electricity of electricity at a quantum degree, we can also loose up new possibilities for healing and transformation. Energy restoration modalities including Reiki, acupuncture, and sound restoration offer tangible methods to address active imbalances and sell regular properly-being. As we keep to discover the quantum perspective of recuperation, we may also additionally find out a deeper expertise of the interconnectedness amongst mind, frame, and electricity, predominant to profound upgrades within the location of healthcare.

Quantum Wellness Techniques for Stress Reduction and Relaxation

In contemporary fast-paced and traumatic world, strain has end up an inevitable a part of our lives. From paintings pressures to personal responsibilities, pressure can take a toll on our physical, intellectual, and emotional well-being. However, with the upgrades in generation and technology, new techniques to stress cut price and rest have emerged. One such approach is quantum properly being techniques, which harness the strength of quantum physics to promote average properly-being. In this text, we're capable of discover the idea of quantum nicely being and delve into a few effective strategies that could help lessen strain and bring about rest.

Quantum health is based totally completely at the necessities of quantum physics, which states that everything within the universe is fabricated from strength. This electricity, additionally called quantum energy, flows thru our bodies and influences our physical, intellectual, and emotional states. Quantum nicely being techniques aim to balance and harmonize this energy, most important to a nation of satisfactory well-being.

One of the maximum famous quantum nicely being strategies for strain discount and rest is quantum meditation. Unlike traditional meditation practices, quantum meditation makes a speciality of gaining access to and harnessing the quantum strength inside us. It involves deep relaxation, visualization, and the use of affirmations to create a fantastic and peaceful nation of thoughts. By tapping into the quantum energy, people can launch stress, beautify popularity, and experience a profound feel of rest.

Another effective approach is quantum respiratory. Breathing is a critical component of our life, and via consciously controlling our breath, we're capable of affect our bodily and intellectual states. Quantum breathing includes sluggish, deep breaths which may be synchronized with best affirmations or visualizations. This approach no longer most effective enables to calm the mind but additionally enhances the waft of quantum energy at some level inside the frame, promoting relaxation and strain cut price.

Quantum properly being techniques also embody the use of quantum crystals and gemstones. Crystals were used for hundreds of years for their recuperation houses, and quantum nicely being takes this idea a step in addition. Each crystal is notion to very personal a totally unique vibrational frequency which can engage with our personal power hassle. By carrying or keeping unique crystals, humans can align their power with the crystal's frequency, selling relaxation and pressure cut fee. For example, amethyst is understood for its calming homes, at the equal time as rose quartz is related to love and emotional healing.

In addition to the ones techniques, quantum well being moreover emphasizes the significance of awesome thinking and purpose putting. Quantum physics shows that our mind and intentions have the strength to influence our reality. By cultivating pleasant thoughts and placing easy intentions for pressure discount and rest, people can create a quantum area of strength that helps their nicely-being. This can be executed via each day affirmations, visualization wearing sports, or maybe growing a imaginative and prescient board that represents their favored country of rest.

Furthermore, quantum nicely-being strategies encourage people to encompass the concept of interconnectedness. Quantum physics shows that the whole lot in the universe is interconnected, and through spotting this interconnectedness, humans can faucet into a extra deliver of power and useful resource. This may be completed via practices which incorporates gratitude, compassion, and mindfulness. By cultivating a experience of gratitude for the prevailing 2nd and showing compassion closer to oneself and others, human beings can create a first rate strength area that promotes rest and strain cut fee.

It is essential to look at that quantum well-being strategies aren't an alternative desire to expert clinical recommendation or remedy. However, they'll be used as complementary practices to resource regular well-being and enhance strain cut charge and relaxation.

In give up, quantum well-being strategies offer a totally particular and effective approach to pressure good deal and relaxation. By harnessing the electricity of quantum physics, people can tap into their private strength field and create a rustic of maximum green well-being. From quantum meditation to quantum breathing, the ones strategies provide sensible tool for dealing with strain and inducing relaxation. By incorporating fine questioning, aim putting, and embracing interconnectedness, people can create a quantum scenario of electricity that lets in their regular nicely-being. So, why not find out the arena of quantum wellness and experience the transformative electricity it holds for stress discount and relaxation?

Healing Modalities: Exploring the Mystical World of Reiki, Acupuncture, and Beyond

In a international wherein cutting-edge-day-day remedy dominates the healthcare panorama, there is a growing interest and hobby in possibility healing modalities. These historic practices, rooted in centuries-vintage traditions, offer a unique mindset on restoration and nicely-being. Among the plethora of alternatives available, Reiki and acupuncture stand out as of the most fascinating and widely practiced modalities.

Let us embark on a journey to find out those charming strategies, in addition to delve into the vicinity of other lesser-recognised healing modalities.

Reiki, a Japanese recuperation approach, has received huge recognition in modern years. The word "Reiki" is derived from Japanese terms: "rei," due to this regular, and "ki," because of this existence stress power. This holistic technique to recovery focuses on channeling this life stress electricity via the practitioner's hands to the recipient, promoting rest, stress discount, and normal well-being. Reiki is primarily based completely at the perception that when the life strain strength is low, we are more prone to contamination and emotional misery. By restoring the stability of this strength, Reiki desires to facilitate the body's natural recovery abilities.

Acupuncture, instead, originates from historic Chinese remedy and is based totally totally completely at the idea of Qi (mentioned "chee"), the vital life pressure that flows through our our our bodies. This modality includes the insertion of skinny needles into unique factors alongside the frame's meridians, or energy pathways, to stimulate the drift of Qi and restore balance. Acupuncture is normally used to alleviate ache, lessen strain, and cope with a massive sort of conditions, together with migraines, digestive problems, or maybe infertility. The exercise of acupuncture is deeply rooted within the perception that imbalances within the body's energy go together with the flow can result in contamination, and with the resource of restoring this stability, health can be regained.

Beyond Reiki and acupuncture, there exists a massive array of lesser-noted restoration modalities that provide particular procedures to nicely-being. One such modality is crystal recovery, which harnesses the energy of numerous crystals and gems to restore balance and sell recovery. Each crystal is notion to very own its very personal unique vibrational frequency, that might engage with our very very own power place, or air of thriller, to bring about physical, emotional, and religious healing. From amethyst, diagnosed for its calming homes, to rose quartz, related to love and compassion, crystals had been used for hundreds of years to enhance everyday properly-being.

Another fascinating restoration modality is sound treatment, which utilizes the energy of sound vibrations to sell restoration and relaxation. Whether thru using making a track bowls, tuning forks, or even the human voice, sound treatment objectives to restore concord in the frame and mind. The vibrations emitted through the ones gadgets are believed to resonate with our personal power, helping to launch blockages, lessen strain, and restore balance. Sound remedy has been used to cope with a large variety of conditions, from anxiety and depression to chronic ache and sleep problems.

A lesser-diagnosed yet in addition charming recuperation modality is aromatherapy, which harnesses the power of critical oils to sell physical and emotional properly-being. These as an opportunity centered plant extracts are believed to own healing houses that can really impact our temper, feelings, and frequently happening fitness. Whether through inhalation, topical software, or even ingestion (underneath the steerage of a expert expert), vital oils may be used to relieve stress, enhance sleep, improve immunity, or maybe enhance cognitive feature. From lavender, recognized for its calming results, to peppermint, famend for its invigorating homes, aromatherapy gives a aromatic and herbal approach to restoration.

Chapter 3: The Power Of Positive Thinking

Understanding Quantum Wellness:

Quantum well being is a holistic approach to nicely-being that integrates ideas from quantum physics, psychology, and spirituality. It recognizes that the whole lot in the universe is interconnected, and that our mind and intentions may want to have an impact at the strength fields round us. This mindset disturbing situations the traditional reductionist view of fitness, emphasizing the want to address the thoughts-body-spirit connection for maximum great nicely-being. Positive wondering serves as a catalyst on this manner, allowing human beings to faucet into the quantum challenge and display up their favored results.

The Power of Positive Thinking:

Positive questioning isn't definitely about adopting a contented disposition or suppressing bad emotions. It is going past floor-degree optimism and delves into the depths of our subconscious thoughts. By cultivating effective thoughts, we are able to rewire our neural pathways, growing new sorts of questioning and behavior. This rewiring approach, known as neuroplasticity, lets in us to break loose from proscribing ideals and self-sabotaging styles, paving the way for private increase and transformation.

The Quantum Mind-Body Connection:

Quantum physics has determined that our mind and intentions have a right away have an effect on on the physical international. The observer impact, a essential precept in quantum mechanics, shows that the act of announcement can alter the behavior of subatomic particles. Similarly, our mind and intentions can shape our bodily reality. Positive wondering, even as combined with centered reason and perception, can activate the frame's innate recuperation mechanisms, selling average properly-being and electricity. This mind-body connection is a powerful tool that may be harnessed to beautify our quantum nicely being.

Authenticity and Originality:

In discussing the power of amazing wondering in quantum well being, it's far vital to emphasise the importance of authenticity and originality. With the proliferation of information inside the virtual age, it is straightforward to fall into the entice of regurgitating thoughts with out inclusive of any unique insights. To certainly discover this problem be counted, we ought to delve into our personal testimonies and views, supplying glowing views and private anecdotes. By doing so, we make contributions to the collective information on quantum nicely-being, fostering a deeper understanding of the problem count number.

Conclusion:

The power of immoderate quality thinking in quantum fitness is a captivating and transformative concept that holds top notch functionality for personal boom and well-being. By spotting the interconnectedness of our mind, emotions, and bodily reality, we're capable of harness the quantum place to reveal up our preferred effects. However, it is vital to technique this concern count with authenticity and originality, contributing to the discourse on quantum properly being in a meaningful and precise manner. By doing so, we're capable of release the proper capability of great thinking and create a harmonious balance between our internal and outer worlds.

Quantum well being and the law of appeal: Manifesting fitness and properly-being

In the huge realm of metaphysics and spirituality, the concept of quantum properly being and the law of enchantment has received big interest. It delves into the profound connection between our thoughts, emotions, and the manifestation of our fitness and properly-being. This captivating ideology shows that via manner of harnessing the strength of our minds and aligning our vibrations with high-quality power, we will appeal to and display up critical fitness and properly-being into our lives.

At the core of this philosophy lies the knowledge that the entirety in the universe, which includes our our bodies, consists of strength. Quantum physics famous that this power is in a ordinary kingdom of vibration, and those vibrations create our truth. The law of enchantment, a vital principle of quantum well being, asserts that like draws like. In other terms, the energy we emit through our mind, emotions, and beliefs attracts corresponding research and results into our lives.

When we observe this principle to our health and nicely-being, we start to understand the large power we preserve inner ourselves. Our mind and feelings have a direct impact on our bodily and highbrow states. Negative mind and feelings can lower our vibrations, major to imbalances and dis-ease inner our our our our bodies. Conversely, fine mind and emotions decorate our vibrations, selling concord and well-being.

To take area health and well-being, we want to first cultivate a deep revel in of self-interest. This includes searching at our mind and feelings, figuring out any horrible styles or restricting beliefs that may be hindering our properly-being. By consciously deciding on to shift our cognizance within the course of wonderful mind and emotions, we're capable of start to reprogram our subconscious mind and align our vibrations with the frequency of fitness and energy.

Visualization and confirmation techniques play a important feature in this manner. By vividly imagining ourselves in a rustic of exceptional health and nicely-being, we prompt the law of enchantment and ship out effective vibrations into the universe. Affirmations, which encompass "I am healthful and colourful," "I trap perfect well-being," or "My frame is a temple of fitness," fortify those first-rate vibrations and rewire our subconscious thoughts to useful resource our desired country of being.

However, it's miles vital to be aware that quantum well-being and the law of enchantment are not an alternative choice to scientific remedy or professional recommendation. They are complementary practices which can beautify our fashionable properly-being and manual the recovery approach. It is critical to are trying to find appropriate sanatorium treatment and make informed choices concerning our fitness.

In forestall, quantum properly being and the regulation of appeal provide a captivating attitude on manifesting fitness and well-being. By understanding the power of our thoughts, emotions, and vibrations, we're able to actively take part in growing our reality. Through self-attention, first-class affirmations, and visualization strategies, we're able to align ourselves with the frequency of most beneficial health and nicely-being. Embracing this philosophy empowers us to take rate of our own nicely-being and embark on a transformative journey towards a vibrant and fulfilling life.

Quantum Wellness and the Mind-Body Connection in Chronic Illness

Understanding Quantum Wellness:

Quantum wellbeing is a holistic approach to health that recognizes the interconnectedness of the mind, body, and spirit. It draws upon standards from quantum physics, which suggests that the whole lot inside the universe is manufactured from electricity and that our thoughts and emotions can impact this power. In the context of chronic infection, quantum fitness acknowledges that our intellectual and emotional states can effect our bodily fitness and vice versa.

The Mind-Body Connection:

The mind-body connection refers to the complicated relationship amongst our thoughts, emotions, and physical properly-being. Research has validated that continual stress, bad feelings, and unresolved trauma can contribute to the development and improvement of persistent illnesses. Conversely, brilliant feelings, a healthy mind-set, and powerful strain manipulate strategies can promote healing and beautify everyday health results.

Harnessing the Power of Thoughts and Emotions:

Quantum well-being emphasizes the significance of cultivating splendid thoughts and feelings to guide restoration in persistent contamination. By consciously directing our thoughts inside the course of optimism, gratitude, and self-compassion, we're capable of create a pleasant energetic environment interior our our our bodies. This remarkable electricity can enhance the frame's herbal restoration mechanisms, enhance the immune gadget, and sell ordinary properly-being.

Practices for Quantum Wellness:

Various practices can assist humans harness the power of quantum nicely-being in persistent infection. Meditation, as an example, permits individuals to quiet the mind, reduce strain, and domesticate a sense of internal peace. Visualization techniques can also be hired to assume the body's cells and organs functioning optimally, promoting recovery at a cellular degree. Additionally, power recovery modalities along with Reiki and acupuncture can help stability the frame's electricity float, facilitating recovery and restoring established nicely being.

The Role of Intuition and Inner Wisdom:

Quantum wellbeing recognizes the significance of intuition and inner expertise in guiding people within the path of most reliable health. By tuning into their internal guidance, people may also want to make informed alternatives approximately their treatment options, way of existence picks, and regular well-being. This intuitive connection can offer valuable insights into the inspiration motives of persistent infection and manual humans within the direction of the most suitable healing modalities.

The Power of Mindfulness:

Mindfulness, the workout of being without a doubt gift in the 2nd, plays a essential function in quantum well-being and the thoughts-frame connection. By cultivating mindfulness, humans can enlarge a deeper recognition of their thoughts, emotions, and bodily sensations. This heightened consciousness lets in for the identification and release of awful concept styles and emotional blockages, promoting healing and restoring balance.

The Importance of Self-Care:

Quantum properly-being emphasizes the importance of self-care in persistent infection. Engaging in sports activities that nourish the mind, frame, and spirit, which encompass regular workout, healthful eating, and engaging in hobbies, can assist everyday properly-being. Additionally, self-care practices which includes journaling, spending time in nature, and connecting with cherished ones can assist human beings manage stress, reduce symptoms and signs, and beautify their notable of life.

Chapter 4: Quantum Wellness

In modern years, the concept of quantum health has obtained giant interest as a holistic technique to attaining universal nicely-being. Quantum wellbeing acknowledges the interconnectedness of the mind, body, and spirit, emphasizing the profound effect that emotions may moreover have on bodily fitness. This particular angle delves into the depths of human existence, exploring the complicated dating among our emotional country and its effect on our physical well-being. By statistics and harnessing this connection, people can unfasten up the functionality for transformative restoration and gain a rustic of finest fitness.

Emotions, often considered intangible and ephemeral, very very own an top notch electricity that extends a long way beyond our conscious recognition. Quantum physics, a department of science that explores the vital nature of reality, offers a framework to realize the complicated workings of emotions and their effect on physical health. According to quantum idea, the whole thing in the universe consists of electricity, collectively with our thoughts, feelings, and bodily our bodies. This energy is constantly in motion, vibrating at precise frequencies, and interconnected with the larger active vicinity that encompasses all of life.

When we experience emotions, whether or no longer nice or horrific, they generate a selected vibrational frequency that resonates at some point of our complete being. These vibrations can have an effect on the energetic stability inside our our bodies, affecting our physical health. For example, persistent pressure, anger, or worry can disrupt the harmonious drift of power, number one to imbalances and ultimately manifesting as bodily ailments. On the opposite hand, emotions which incorporates love, satisfaction, and gratitude can decorate the vibrational frequency, selling restoration and everyday well-being.

The impact of feelings on physical health may be located through numerous medical studies and anecdotal proof. Research has proven that continual strain, as an instance, can weaken the immune device, growth the danger of cardiovascular diseases, and make contributions to the development of intellectual health problems. Similarly, terrible feelings like anger and resentment were related to extended infection within the body, it's associated with a sizeable shape of continual conditions, in conjunction with autoimmune ailments, diabetes, or maybe most cancers.

Conversely, exceptional feelings were positioned to have a profound effect on bodily fitness. Studies have proven that people who experience emotions consisting of affection, compassion, and happiness have a tendency to have lower blood stress, reduced degrees of stress hormones, and a stronger immune device. Moreover, cultivating super feelings has been related to improved cognitive function, greater suitable sturdiness, and a higher famous excellent of lifestyles.

Understanding the connection among feelings and bodily health opens up a global of opportunities for healing and nicely-being. By acknowledging and addressing our emotional usa, we are capable of actively take part in our private healing gadget. This involves developing emotional intelligence, which encompasses the ability to understand, recognize, and control our emotions efficaciously. Through practices which includes mindfulness, meditation, and self-meditated picture, we are able to cultivate emotional resilience and create a high high-quality inner surroundings that facilitates our physical health.

Furthermore, quantum health encourages human beings to find out the concept motives in their feelings and deal with them at a deeper diploma. Emotions are regularly a reflection of our beliefs, beyond research, and unconscious programming. By delving into those underlying factors, we turns into privy to and release emotional blockages that may be hindering our physical properly-being. This method of emotional restoration can involve diverse recovery modalities, in conjunction with psychotherapy, strength recuperation, and somatic practices, which goal to restore balance and harmony within the thoughts-frame tool.

In end, quantum well-being gives a unique angle on the effect of feelings on bodily fitness. By spotting the interconnectedness of our emotional and physical states, we are able to harness the transformative electricity of our feelings to acquire maximum high-quality properly-being. Through practices that domesticate emotional intelligence and address the inspiration motives of our feelings, we are able to create a harmonious inner environment that helps our physical fitness. Embracing the concepts of quantum wellbeing permits us to embark on a adventure of self-discovery and recovery, unlocking the ability for a colorful and satisfying lifestyles.

Quantum Wellness Practices for Enhancing Mental Clarity and Focus

Understanding Quantum Wellness:

Quantum well being is a holistic method that combines requirements from quantum physics, spirituality, and nicely-being practices to promote preferred nicely-being. It recognizes that the whole lot inside the universe is interconnected and that our mind and intentions have a profound impact on our reality. Quantum nicely being practices aim to align our mind, emotions, and actions with our preferred results, permitting us to tap into the limitless capability of the quantum region.

Enhancing Mental Clarity and Focus thru Quantum Wellness Practices:

1. Mindfulness Meditation:

Mindfulness meditation is a effective practice that cultivates present-2d interest and enhances intellectual clarity and recognition. By focusing on the breath and looking at thoughts with out judgment, people can educate their minds to live centered and decrease intellectual chatter. This workout has been scientifically mounted to increase gray depend inside the mind, enhance cognitive function, and decrease pressure levels.

2. Visualization and Affirmations:

Visualization and affirmations are strategies that leverage the power of the thoughts to seem preferred consequences. By vividly imagining oneself in a rustic of mental readability and interest, individuals can reprogram their subconscious thoughts and align their thoughts with their intentions. Affirmations, collectively with "I am centered and clean-minded," can give a boost to extraordinary ideals and decorate intellectual clarity.

3. Energy Healing:

Energy recuperation modalities, together with Reiki and acupuncture, paintings at the principle that strength flows through the frame and affects frequently occurring properly-being. By clearing lively blockages and balancing the body's strength centers, people can revel in progressed mental readability and attention. These practices sell relaxation, lessen pressure, and enhance the body's herbal recuperation abilties.

4. Quantum Entrainment:

Quantum entrainment is a way that uses the power of aim and resonance to synchronize brainwave patterns and decorate intellectual readability and interest. By paying attention to particular frequencies or the usage of binaural beats, human beings can entrain their brainwaves to a preferred kingdom, which incorporates alpha or theta, which can be associated with heightened consciousness and creativity. This practice can be specially beneficial at some point of meditation or while carrying out mentally stressful duties.

5. Nutritional Support:

Proper vitamins performs a critical function in keeping primary mind feature and enhancing mental readability and interest. Consuming a balanced weight loss program rich in antioxidants, omega-three fatty acids, and vitamins B and D can aid mind health and enhance cognitive feature. Additionally, incorporating mind-boosting food, which include blueberries, walnuts, and dark chocolate, can offer a herbal cognitive improve.

6. Physical Exercise:

Regular physical exercising has been tested to have numerous advantages for mental readability and consciousness. Exercise will increase blood drift to the mind, promotes the release of endorphins, and improves regular cognitive feature. Engaging in sports which includes yoga, tai chi, or cardio exercise can decorate intellectual readability, reduce strain, and beautify reputation.

Conclusion:

In end, quantum properly being practices provide a unique and effective technique to decorate highbrow clarity and popularity. By incorporating mindfulness meditation, visualization, energy restoration, quantum entrainment, right vitamins, and physical exercise into our every day workout routines, we're able to faucet into our innate functionality and benefit a state of heightened intellectual clarity and popularity. These practices no longer best sell common well-being but moreover empower people to navigate the challenges of current life correctly and appeal. Embracing the mind of quantum health can result in a profound transformation in our highbrow, emotional, and spiritual nicely-being, allowing us to stay a lifestyles of readability, attention, and fulfillment.

Quantum Wellness Practices for Enhancing Mental Clarity and Focus

Understanding Quantum Wellness:

Quantum fitness is a holistic method that combines necessities from quantum physics, spirituality, and nicely being practices to sell everyday properly-being. It recognizes that the whole lot inside the universe is interconnected and that our mind and intentions have a profound effect on our fact. Quantum nicely-being practices reason to align our mind, feelings, and movements with our preferred results, allowing us to tap into the endless ability of the quantum subject.

Enhancing Mental Clarity and Focus through Quantum Wellness Practices:

1. Mindfulness Meditation:

Mindfulness meditation is a powerful workout that cultivates present-2d interest and complements intellectual clarity and attention. By focusing on the breath and watching thoughts without judgment, humans can teach their minds to live centered and decrease highbrow chatter. This exercising has been scientifically hooked up to boom grey rely within the thoughts, enhance cognitive feature, and decrease stress levels.

2. Visualization and Affirmations:

Visualization and affirmations are techniques that leverage the strength of the mind to occur preferred outcomes. By vividly imagining oneself in a kingdom of intellectual readability and consciousness, human beings can reprogram their unconscious mind and align their thoughts with their intentions. Affirmations, collectively with "I am focused and smooth-minded," can aid excellent ideals and decorate highbrow readability.

three. Energy Healing:

Energy recovery modalities, together with Reiki and acupuncture, artwork at the principle that energy flows via the frame and impacts simple properly-being. By clearing lively blockages and balancing the frame's strength facilities, humans can experience improved highbrow clarity and interest. These practices promote rest, lessen strain, and enhance the body's herbal recovery abilities.

4. Quantum Entrainment:

Quantum entrainment is a way that uses the energy of intention and resonance to synchronize brainwave styles and beautify intellectual readability and popularity. By being attentive to unique frequencies or the usage of binaural beats, human beings can entrain their brainwaves to a favored state, alongside aspect alpha or theta, which might be associated with heightened focus and creativity. This workout may be specifically beneficial at some point of meditation or while carrying out mentally disturbing obligations.

5. Nutritional Support:

Proper vitamins plays a critical function in preserving most effective mind characteristic and improving intellectual clarity and attention. Consuming a balanced eating regimen wealthy in antioxidants, omega-three fatty acids, and vitamins B and D can help mind fitness and beautify cognitive function. Additionally, incorporating thoughts-boosting food, along side blueberries, walnuts, and dark chocolate, can offer a natural cognitive decorate.

6. Physical Exercise:

Regular bodily exercise has been tested to have severa blessings for mental clarity and interest. Exercise will increase blood glide to the mind, promotes the discharge of endorphins, and improves common cognitive feature. Engaging in sports activities along with yoga, tai chi, or aerobic exercising can beautify intellectual clarity, reduce strain, and enhance attention.

Conclusion:

In cease, quantum health practices offer a very particular and powerful technique to enhance highbrow clarity and consciousness.

By incorporating mindfulness meditation, visualization, energy restoration, quantum entrainment, right nutrients, and physical exercising into our every day sporting activities, we can faucet into our innate capability and advantage a state of heightened highbrow clarity and popularity. These practices not satisfactory promote commonplace well-being but moreover empower people to navigate the demanding situations of present day life without problem and allure. Embracing the thoughts of quantum well being can result in a profound transformation in our intellectual, emotional, and spiritual well-being, allowing us to live a lifestyles of clarity, attention, and success.

Chapter 5: Nourishing The Mind And Body

In the pursuit of normal nicely-being, its miles essential to apprehend the profound effect that nutrients has on our mind and body. The idea of quantum properly-being emphasizes the interconnectedness of all factors of our being, together with physical, highbrow, and religious health. Nutrition plays a pivotal position in attaining this country of holistic nicely-being, as it provides the essential gas and building blocks for our our bodies and minds to thrive.

The mind-frame connection is a essential precept in quantum well being. Our highbrow and emotional states are intricately related to our physical fitness, and vitamins acts as a catalyst for this connection. When we nourish our our bodies with wholesome, nutrient-dense foods, we offer the essential basis for max extraordinary thoughts characteristic and emotional well-being.

One of the important element techniques nutrients impacts our highbrow fitness is through the manufacturing of neurotransmitters. These chemical messengers play a crucial position in regulating our temper, cognition, and ordinary mental country. For instance, serotonin, often known as the "revel in-proper" neurotransmitter, is synthesized from the amino acid tryptophan, this is decided in protein-wealthy food. By ingesting a balanced healthy dietweight-reduction plan that consists of property of tryptophan, which consist of turkey, eggs, and nuts, we will assist the manufacturing of serotonin and promote a extremely good intellectual u . S . A ..

Furthermore, nutrients plays a essential function in maintaining cognitive characteristic and preventing age-associated decline. The thoughts calls for a consistent supply of vitamins, along with omega-three fatty acids, antioxidants, and vitamins, to function optimally. Omega-3 fatty acids, observed in fatty fish like salmon and walnuts, were validated to beautify cognitive universal performance and protect in competition to cognitive decline. Antioxidants, enough in colorful culmination and greens, help fight oxidative pressure and infection, which can be implicated in neurodegenerative illnesses like Alzheimer's. By incorporating those nutrient-rich components into our diets, we are capable of nourish our minds and assist lengthy-time period thoughts fitness.

In addition to its effect on highbrow health, nutrients moreover performs a important characteristic in physical well-being. The food we devour serves due to the fact the constructing blocks for our our bodies, imparting the important vitamins for increase, repair, and preservation. A food plan rich in complete meals, which includes lean proteins, whole grains, culmination, and greens, substances the important nutrients, minerals, and macronutrients desired for top of the road bodily characteristic.

Protein, for example, is a important nutrient for muscle increase and repair. It gives the critical amino acids for the synthesis of latest muscle organizations and aids inside the restoration approach after physical interest. Incorporating lean assets of protein, which encompass chicken, fish, and legumes, into our diets can guide muscle improvement and ordinary bodily energy.

Furthermore, proper nutrients is crucial for preserving a healthful weight and stopping continual illnesses. Obesity, a developing worldwide health concern, is mostly a end result of negative dietary alternatives and an imbalance amongst strength intake and expenditure. By adopting a balanced and nutrient-dense weight loss plan, we're capable of help weight manage and decrease the danger of situations such as diabetes, cardiovascular ailment, and positive styles of most cancers.

Moreover, vitamins performs a large function in assisting our immune gadget, it genuinely is critical for defensive in opposition to pathogens and preserving everyday fitness. A nicely-nourished body is better ready to fight off infections and get over ailments. Key nutrients, collectively with vitamins C, nutrients D, zinc, and probiotics, play a important feature in supporting immune characteristic. Citrus give up result, leafy greens, dairy merchandise, and fermented food are exceptional property of those immune-boosting vitamins.

In the arena of quantum well being, nutrients extends past the physical and intellectual factors of our properly-being. It also encompasses the non secular size, due to the reality the food we consume also can have a profound impact on our spiritual increase and connection to the area around us. Many spiritual traditions emphasize the importance of aware ingesting, in which people cultivate a deep interest and gratitude for the food they consume.

By strolling toward conscious eating, we are able to develop a extra profound connection to the meals we devour, recognizing the energy and life pressure it provides. This reputation permits us to make conscious picks about the meals we eat, choosing folks who align with our values and guide our primary nicely-being. Whether it is selecting herbal, regionally sourced produce or embracing a plant-based totally food regimen for moral motives, nutrients becomes a automobile for non secular increase and alignment with our higher selves.

In end, the function of vitamins in quantum well being is multifaceted and profound. It nourishes our minds and our our our bodies, supporting maximum pleasant mind characteristic, emotional properly-being, and cognitive health. Nutrition moreover performs a crucial function in bodily properly-being, presenting the critical vitamins for increase, repair, and protection. Furthermore, it extends to the non secular size, permitting us to cultivate a deeper connection to the meals we eat and align our nutritional picks with our values. By recognizing the power of nutrients in accomplishing holistic fitness, we're able to embark on a adventure of self-discovery and transformation, nourishing each our minds and bodies for a vibrant and fun life.

Quantum Wellness and the Importance of Sleep for Overall Well-being

In the short-paced world we stay in, in which technology has become an crucial a part of our lives, it is easy to overlook the significance of sleep for our everyday nicely-being. However, cutting-edge clinical research has shed mild on the profound impact that sleep has on our physical, highbrow, and emotional fitness. In the sector of quantum fitness, sleep performs a critical function in conducting a state of balance and concord within ourselves.

Quantum nicely being is a holistic method to properly-being that acknowledges the interconnectedness of our mind, frame, and spirit. It recognizes that we aren't simply bodily beings, however additionally active beings, and that our properly-being is influenced with the resource of the diffused energies that go with the flow via us. Sleep, in this context, is seen as a vital detail of preserving and improving the ones energies.

When we sleep, our our our bodies go through a chain of complex strategies which can be important for our preferred fitness. During sleep, our cells regenerate, our immune system strengthens, and our mind consolidates reminiscences and techniques feelings. Without enough sleep, those strategies are disrupted, principal to loads of poor consequences for our nicely-being.

One of the maximum huge impacts of sleep deprivation is on our cognitive characteristic. Lack of sleep impairs our functionality to pay interest, make picks, and treatment issues. It moreover affects our reminiscence, making it difficult to hold facts and studies new topics. In a global that desires normal mental agility, the importance of sleep for cognitive nicely-being cannot be overstated.

Furthermore, sleep deprivation has a profound impact on our emotional properly-being. Studies have proven that sleep-deprived humans are more likely to enjoy mood swings, irritability, and heightened emotional reactivity. This can strain relationships, prevent powerful conversation, and bring about a large revel in of dissatisfaction and unhappiness. Sleep, therefore, acts as a foundation for emotional stability and resilience.

Chapter 6: The Benefits Of Regular Exercise

In trendy speedy-paced and worrying international, attaining a rustic of wellbeing is turning into increasingly critical. Quantum properly being, a holistic method to fitness and recovery, recognizes the interconnectedness of the thoughts, body, and spirit. It emphasizes the significance of maintaining stability and concord in all elements of life. Regular exercising is a key component of quantum fitness, as it gives severa advantages for each the thoughts and body, promoting regular properly-being and facilitating the restoration tool.

Exercise has lengthy been recognized for its bodily advantages, collectively with weight management, improved cardiovascular fitness, and extended electricity and versatility. However, its effect on mental and emotional well-being is frequently omitted. Engaging in regular physical interest releases endorphins, the frame's natural sense-actual chemical materials, that may assist alleviate signs of depression, tension, and strain. Exercise moreover will boom the production of serotonin and dopamine, neurotransmitters that play a important feature in regulating temper and promoting a enjoy of happiness and properly-being.

Moreover, ordinary exercising has been showed to enhance cognitive feature and enhance mental clarity. Physical hobby will increase blood go along with the go with the flow to the mind, delivering oxygen and vitamins which might be critical for best mind characteristic. It also stimulates the release of boom elements, which sell the formation of latest neurons and connections in the mind, improving memory, focus, and common cognitive overall performance. In reality, research have shown that people who have interplay in regular workout have a discounted hazard of growing cognitive decline and neurodegenerative illnesses, in conjunction with Alzheimer's and Parkinson's.

In addition to its intellectual and physical advantages, exercise is a powerful tool for mind-frame restoration. Quantum wellness acknowledges that the thoughts and frame are interconnected, and that addressing one's emotional and intellectual well-being is important for reaching principal health. Regular exercising offers a completely unique possibility to connect to one's frame, fostering a deeper enjoy of self-recognition and selling a high-quality frame photo. It allows human beings to song in to their bodily sensations, feelings, and mind, growing a area for self-mirrored photo and self-discovery.

Furthermore, exercising can feature a shape of meditation, permitting humans to quiet their minds and find internal peace. Engaging in sports activities which include yoga, tai chi, or aware walking can help domesticate a kingdom of mindfulness, in which one is actually gift within the moment and attuned to their body and surroundings. This exercise of mindfulness no longer best reduces strain and tension however additionally promotes a experience of connectedness and group spirit with the universe, aligning with the standards of quantum nicely being.

Regular workout furthermore performs a critical characteristic within the frame's herbal healing strategies. Physical hobby stimulates the lymphatic device, that is responsible for eliminating pollution and waste merchandise from the body. By growing lymphatic go with the flow, exercising permits to decorate the immune device, enhancing the body's capability to fight off infections and ailments. It additionally promotes the manufacturing of endorphins, which act as natural painkillers, lowering ache and selling quicker restoration from injuries or illnesses.

Moreover, exercising has been showed to have a incredible impact at the frame's strain reaction device. Chronic strain should have detrimental results on each the thoughts and frame, number one to a tremendous style of health problems, which includes cardiovascular ailment, digestive troubles, and highbrow fitness issues. Regular exercise permits to adjust the body's pressure hormones, at the side of cortisol, and promotes the discharge of endorphins, which counteract the horrible outcomes of stress. This now not handiest improves regular nicely-being however moreover strengthens the body's resilience to destiny stressors.

In cease, quantum wellness recognizes the importance of keeping stability and concord in all elements of life, collectively with the mind, frame, and spirit. Regular exercising is a effective device for achieving this stability, providing numerous benefits for every the mind and frame. It promotes intellectual and emotional properly-being, complements cognitive characteristic, and allows mind-body recuperation. By challenge ordinary physical pastime, human beings can revel in improved temper, decreased stress and tension, progressed self-consciousness, and a more experience of normal nicely-being. Embracing the standards of quantum properly-being and incorporating ordinary exercising into one's lifestyle can motive a profound transformation and a deeper reference to oneself and the arena round us.

Exploring the Role of Meditation and Mindfulness in Quantum Wellness

Understanding Quantum Wellness:

Quantum nicely being is a holistic approach to nicely-being that acknowledges the interconnectedness of all factors of our being – bodily, highbrow, emotional, and spiritual. It attracts perception from the standards of quantum physics, which advocate that the whole thing in the universe is interconnected and stimulated through the use of our mind and intentions. Quantum fitness emphasizes the energy of our hobby and the function it plays in shaping our truth.

Meditation and Mindfulness:

Meditation and mindfulness are historic practices that have been used for masses of years to cultivate a state of internal peace and self-interest. Meditation consists of focusing one's interest and doing away with the glide of mind that continuously occupy our minds. Mindfulness, however, involves being truly gift in the 2nd, searching at our mind and feelings with out judgment.

Both meditation and mindfulness are powerful tool for quieting the mind, decreasing stress, and improving average well-being. They allow us to faucet into our internal knowledge and hook up with our authentic selves. By running within the route of meditation and mindfulness, we're able to domesticate a experience of internal calm and readability, permitting us to navigate lifestyles's stressful situations with extra ease and resilience.

The Quantum Connection:

Quantum physics suggests that at the maximum crucial level, everything inside the universe is made up of strength. Our mind and intentions also are types of electricity, and that they have got the energy to persuade the world round us. By jogging in the direction of meditation and mindfulness, we are capable of harness the electricity of our consciousness to shape our fact and create top notch change in our lives.

Quantum health recognizes that our mind and emotions have a right away effect on our bodily and intellectual well-being. Negative thoughts and emotions can create energetic blockages in our our our bodies, primary to bodily illnesses and emotional imbalances. By cultivating a rustic of mindfulness and running closer to meditation, we are capable of release these energetic blockages and repair stability to our our bodies and minds.

The Benefits of Meditation and Mindfulness in Quantum Wellness:

1. Stress Reduction: Meditation and mindfulness had been scientifically set up to lessen strain stages by means of way of way of activating the body's rest reaction. By training those techniques often, we are able to decrease our cortisol ranges, enhance our

immune characteristic, and decorate our tremendous well-being.

2. Emotional Balance: Meditation and mindfulness help us develop a more sense of self-attention and emotional intelligence. By looking at our thoughts and emotions with out judgment, we're able to advantage perception into our patterns of questioning and reacting. This allows us to reply to difficult situations with greater clarity and compassion.

3. Improved Focus and Concentration: Regular meditation and mindfulness exercising had been showed to enhance cognitive function, inclusive of attention, consciousness, and reminiscence. By education our minds to live gift and focused, we are able to improve our productiveness and common performance in numerous regions of lifestyles.

four. Enhanced Intuition and Creativity: Meditation and mindfulness open the door to our instinct and creativity. By quieting the thoughts and connecting with our internal cognizance, we will faucet into new mind, insights, and answers to issues.

5. Physical Healing: Quantum fitness recognizes the thoughts-body connection and the feature of interest in physical restoration. By practicing meditation and mindfulness, we are capable of set off the body's natural recuperation mechanisms and promote ordinary properly-being.

Conclusion:

In stop, meditation and mindfulness play a important function in quantum properly-being thru harnessing the energy of our interest to form our fact and decorate our well-being. By training the ones strategies, we are capable of reduce stress, domesticate emotional balance, enhance interest and attention, enhance instinct and creativity, and sell physical healing. Quantum well being invitations us to find out the interconnectedness of all elements of our being and recognize the profound effect our mind and intentions have on our lives. By integrating meditation and mindfulness into our every day lives, we're capable of embark on a transformative adventure closer to holistic well-being.

Quantum Wellness and the Power of Visualization for Healing: Unleashing the Potential Within

The Quantum Nature of Wellness:

Quantum physics famous that on the most critical degree, the whole thing inside the universe consists of power. This energy is in a normal u.S. Of flux, vibrating at special frequencies. Our mind and feelings also emit energy, that could have an effect on the active field spherical us. Quantum health acknowledges that our mind and beliefs form our fact, and by means of manner of consciously directing our mind, we can have an effect on our well-being.

Visualization: A Gateway to Quantum Healing:

Visualization is a powerful approach that lets in us to tap into the quantum realm and harness the power internal. By growing vivid intellectual pics of our desired consequences, we align our thoughts and emotions with the frequency of what we need to reveal up. Visualization turns on the current power of the thoughts, stimulating the unconscious to artwork towards accomplishing our dreams. It serves as a bridge a few of the aware and subconscious thoughts, allowing us to reprogram proscribing ideals and free up our innate recuperation functionality.

The Mind-Body Connection:

The thoughts-body connection is a vital element of quantum health. Scientific studies has tested that our mind and emotions right away impact our bodily health. Negative thoughts and strain can seem as bodily illnesses, while first-rate mind and emotions can sell healing and well-being. Visualization acts as a catalyst for this mind-frame connection, allowing us to direct our thoughts closer to restoration and restoration.

The Power of Intention:

Intention is a key thing of visualization. By setting clean intentions, we align our recognition and strength inside the course of a specific final outcomes. When combined with visualization, reason amplifies the energy of our thoughts, growing a robust pressure for healing. By visualizing our favored united states of properly being and preserving the motive for its manifestation, we faucet into the quantum area and invite healing energies to go along with the go with the flow via us.

The Role of Emotions:

Emotions play a important position inside the technique of visualization for healing. When we visualize, it's miles crucial to evoke the corresponding effective feelings related to our favored outcome. Emotions act as a catalyst, amplifying the vibrational frequency of our thoughts and intentions. By infusing our visualizations with love, gratitude, and joy, we create a harmonious resonance that attracts recovery energies and speeds up the manifestation way.

The Quantum Observer Effect:

The observer impact, a principle in quantum physics, states that the act of commentary affects the behavior of particles. Similarly, our targeted attention and notion within the energy of visualization may have an effect on the very last outcomes of our recuperation journey. By becoming aware observers of our thoughts and actively accomplishing visualization, we emerge as active contributors in our private recuperation machine. We shift from being passive recipients of remedy to empowered co-creators of our properly-being.

Conclusion:

Quantum fitness and the electricity of visualization for recovery provide a profound knowledge of the interconnectedness among our thoughts, feelings, and bodily nicely-being. By harnessing the ideas of quantum physics, we're capable of tap into the infinite capacity internal us. Visualization serves as a gateway to this capacity, allowing us to reprogram our beliefs, align our intentions, and get up our desired state of nicely being. By embracing the power of visualization, we embark on a transformative journey toward holistic restoration, unlocking the quantum nature of our lifestyles.

Chapter 7: Environmental Factors On Health

Understanding Environmental Factors:

Environmental elements encompass a massive variety of factors that surround us, on the aspect of physical, social, and mental additives. These factors can appreciably affect our health, either definitely or negatively. Physical environmental factors together with air and water first-rate, publicity to pollution, and access to green regions can at once impact our bodily properly-being. Social environmental factors, collectively with our relationships, network assist, and socioeconomic reputation, can have an effect on our highbrow and emotional fitness. Lastly, intellectual environmental factors, collectively with stress stages, mindset, and perception systems, can profoundly have an effect on our common properly being.

The Interplay among Quantum Wellness and Environmental Factors:

Quantum health recognizes that our fitness isn't totally decided thru our genetics or person alternatives but is deeply intertwined with the surroundings wherein we stay. It recognizes that we're energetic beings continuously interacting with our surroundings. By embracing this perspective, we're able to better recognize how environmental elements can form our well-being and take proactive steps to optimize our health.

Physical Environmental Factors:

The physical environment we inhabit performs a essential function in our fitness. Air pollutants, as an instance, has been related to respiration illnesses, cardiovascular troubles, or maybe cognitive impairments. Quantum well being encourages us to remember of the air we breathe and take measures to decorate indoor air remarkable through right air drift, air purifiers, and the use of herbal cleaning products. Similarly, water brilliant is essential for our regular nicely-being. Quantum fitness prompts us to be conscious of the water we consume and do not forget making an investment in water filtration systems to reduce publicity to risky contaminants.

Furthermore, get right of entry to to inexperienced regions and publicity to nature have been confirmed to have numerous fitness benefits. Quantum well being encourages us to spend time in herbal environments, as it could reduce strain, enhance mood, and beautify time-honored strength. By incorporating nature into our each day lives, whether or not or not or no longer via gardening, trekking, or absolutely taking a stroll in the park, we are capable of harness the healing energy of the surroundings.

Social Environmental Factors:

Our social environment profoundly influences our highbrow and emotional well-being. Quantum well-being emphasizes the importance of cultivating awesome relationships and a supportive community. Research has usually confirmed that people with sturdy social connections enjoy higher intellectual fitness, lower expenses of persistent sicknesses, and expanded durability. Quantum properly-being encourages us to foster large connections, engage in social sports activities activities, and are looking for for help even as desired. By nurturing our social surroundings, we are able to create a basis for number one properly-being.

Socioeconomic popularity is some other important social environmental detail that impacts health results. Quantum fitness recognizes the disparities that exist in society and calls for collective movement to deal with those inequalities. By advocating for equitable get right of entry to to healthcare, education, and resources, we are capable of create a more inclusive and supportive surroundings for all people to thrive.

Psychological Environmental Factors:

Our attitude, beliefs, and stress degrees substantially impact our health. Quantum nicely-being acknowledges the electricity of our mind and emotions in shaping our well-being. Stress, whether from artwork, relationships, or particular sources, ought to have damaging effects on our physical and highbrow fitness. Quantum properly being encourages us to boom effective strain control strategies, along with meditation, mindfulness, and relaxation sports activities sports. By cultivating a tremendous thoughts-set and adopting wholesome coping mechanisms, we are able to mitigate the horrible impact of strain on our well-being.

Moreover, our notion structures and attitudes inside the path of fitness play a essential function in our popular wellness. Quantum fitness promotes a holistic approach to fitness, encouraging us to view our our bodies as interconnected systems and to do not forget possibility treatments and practices that complement traditional treatment. By embracing a more expansive attitude on fitness, we will tap into the electricity of our thoughts-body connection and decorate our well-being.

Conclusion:

In conclusion, quantum fitness gives a very unique and holistic approach to records and optimizing our fitness. By recognizing the profound impact of environmental elements on our nicely-being, we're able to take proactive steps to create a extra wholesome and further balanced life. Whether it's miles addressing physical environmental elements, nurturing our social connections, or cultivating a first-rate attitude, quantum health empowers us to encompass our interconnectedness with the environment and harness its restoration functionality. By integrating the principles of quantum nicely-being into our lives, we're capable of embark on a transformative journey in the course of maximum appropriate fitness and properly-being.

Quantum Wellness and the Role of Spirituality in Mind-Body Healing

In modern-day rapid-paced and demanding worldwide, the concept of fitness has taken on a whole new this means that. It is not pretty a good deal physical health, but furthermore about reaching a rustic of balance and concord in all elements of our lives. Quantum health, a term coined thru writer and nicely-being expert Kathy Freston, takes this concept a step similarly by way of using incorporating the necessities of quantum physics and spirituality into the area of thoughts-body recovery. This holistic technique recognizes the interconnectedness of our bodily, intellectual, emotional, and religious nicely-being, and emphasizes the feature of spirituality in reaching maximum useful fitness and recovery.

At its center, quantum well being is primarily based at the requirements of quantum physics, which states that the whole thing in the universe is crafted from energy and interconnected via a web of vibrations. This consists of our thoughts, emotions, and beliefs, which may be all forms of electricity that may effect our physical fitness and well-being. Quantum fitness acknowledges that our thoughts and feelings have a right away impact on our bodily our our our bodies, and that with the aid of using moving our electricity and mind-set, we're able to sell recovery and nicely-being on a deep diploma.

Spirituality performs a crucial feature in quantum health, because it gives a framework for expertise and connecting with the higher additives of ourselves and the universe. It is thru spirituality that we are able to tap into our internal expertise, instinct, and better awareness, which are vital for healing and transformation. Spirituality allows us to transcend the limitations of the physical international and get proper of entry to a deeper level of reputation and know-how.

One of the key factors of spirituality in mind-body recovery is the belief in a higher energy or commonplace intelligence. This belief acknowledges that there can be a more force at work in the universe, and that we're all associated with this divine energy. By aligning ourselves with this better strength, we are able to faucet into its recuperation strength and attain steerage and assist on our recuperation journey.

Chapter 8: The Connection Among Gut Health

In modern years, there has been a developing hobby within the idea of quantum health, which emphasizes the interconnectedness of the mind, frame, and spirit. This holistic method to well-being recognizes that our bodily health is deeply intertwined with our highbrow and emotional states. One vicinity that has obtained vast hobby on this regard is the relationship amongst gut health and fundamental well-being. Emerging studies suggests that the health of our intestine microbiome, the complex environment of microorganisms living in our digestive tract, performs a essential position in maintaining maximum right bodily and highbrow health. Understanding this connection and taking steps to decorate gut fitness might also additionally have profound implications for our general nicely-being.

The intestine microbiome, which consist of trillions of bacteria, viruses, fungi, and different microorganisms, is frequently referred to as our "second thoughts." This is because it communicates bidirectionally with our critical worried tool thru a complex network of nerves, hormones, and immune cells. This verbal exchange pathway, known as the gut-brain axis, lets in the gut microbiome to persuade our mood, cognition, and conduct, at the same time as moreover being inspired through our mind and emotions. The complicated dating a number of the gut and the thoughts highlights the importance of maintaining a wholesome gut microbiome for fashionable nicely-being.

One of the essential issue elements influencing gut health is the range and stability of the gut microbiome. A numerous microbiome, with a huge sort of useful bacteria, is associated with higher not unusual fitness. On the other hand, an imbalance in the intestine microbiome, known as dysbiosis, has been connected to some of fitness issues, which include digestive problems, autoimmune ailments, obesity, and highbrow health troubles which encompass tension and depression. Therefore, nurturing a numerous and balanced intestine microbiome is vital for promoting maximum applicable nicely-being.

Several elements can effect the composition and variety of the intestine microbiome. Diet performs a critical characteristic, as certain ingredients can each sell the boom of beneficial micro organism or disrupt the steadiness of the microbiome. A food plan wealthy in fiber, fruits, veggies, and fermented substances offers the critical vitamins for the increase of useful micro organism, whilst a healthy dietweight-reduction plan immoderate in processed components, sugar, and awful fats can negatively impact the microbiome. Therefore, adopting a wholesome and balanced diet is a critical step toward improving gut fitness and standard properly-being.

In addition to weight loss program, specific manner of lifestyles factors can also have an impact on gut health. Chronic stress, for example, has been set up to disrupt the stability of the intestine microbiome, primary to contamination and prolonged susceptibility to severa illnesses. Engaging in strain-reducing practices which includes meditation, yoga, and ordinary exercise can assist restore stability to the gut microbiome and sell regular properly-being. Furthermore, suitable enough sleep is essential for keeping a healthful gut microbiome, as sleep deprivation has been proven to regulate the composition of the microbiome and increase the chance of numerous health troubles.

The connection between gut fitness and everyday well-being extends beyond physical health. Emerging research shows that the gut microbiome additionally performs a function in highbrow health and emotional nicely-being. The intestine-thoughts axis allows the gut microbiome to supply neurotransmitters and different molecules which have an impact on mood and cognition. For instance, excellent strains of bacteria within the intestine produce serotonin, a neurotransmitter called the "experience-appropriate" hormone. Imbalances in the intestine microbiome have been linked to intellectual health troubles on the aspect of anxiety and depression. Therefore, enhancing gut health may additionally have a top notch effect on intellectual and emotional nicely-being.

In surrender, the concept of quantum well being emphasizes the interconnectedness of numerous elements of our well-being, which encompass the relationship between intestine health and not unusual nicely-being. The gut microbiome, regularly referred to as our "second thoughts," performs a essential characteristic in maintaining maximum suitable bodily and intellectual fitness. Nurturing a various and balanced intestine microbiome thru a wholesome food plan, strain cut price, normal workout, and unique sufficient sleep is important for promoting everyday well-being. By recognizing and addressing the relationship among gut fitness and common nicely-being, we are able to embark on a journey in the direction of quantum wellness, in which our thoughts, body, and spirit are in concord, essential to a greater colorful and gratifying existence.

Quantum Wellness Practices for Boosting the Immune System

Understanding Quantum Wellness:

Quantum fitness is a holistic technique to properly-being that draws idea from quantum physics, which explores the vital nature of truth at the subatomic diploma. It acknowledges that everything inside the universe is interconnected and that our mind, feelings, and ideals have a profound impact on our physical fitness. Quantum nicely-being practices goal to align our energy fields, enhance our vibrational frequencies, and promote everyday well-being.

The Immune System and Quantum Wellness:

The immune machine is a complicated network of cells, tissues, and organs that paintings together to shield the frame in the direction of volatile invaders. Quantum fitness practices can notably have an effect on the immune tool's functioning by manner of addressing the underlying active imbalances that would compromise its effectiveness. By promoting a harmonious go with the glide of electricity at some point of the frame, quantum health practices can optimize immune responses and beautify our herbal defense mechanisms.

1. Mind-Body Connection:

Quantum well-being acknowledges the effective connection most of the mind and frame. Our thoughts and feelings can each help or prevent our immune device's functioning. Negative mind and strain can weaken the immune device, at the same time as high high-quality thoughts and feelings can enhance its effectiveness. Quantum nicely being practices, such as meditation, visualization, and terrific affirmations, can assist reprogram our minds, reduce strain, and promote a exquisite outlook, thereby boosting our immune gadget.

2. Energy Healing:

Quantum nicely-being consists of numerous strength recuperation modalities that might honestly impact the immune device. Practices like Reiki, acupuncture, and sound treatment paintings at the precept of restoring the body's strength go with the float and getting rid of lively blockages. By balancing the frame's strength facilities, known as chakras, the ones practices can enhance the immune device's functioning and promote common well-being.

three. Quantum Nutrition:

Quantum nicely being emphasizes the importance of nutrients in assisting immune fitness. Quantum nutrients makes a speciality of eating high-vibrational food which can be rich in important vitamins, antioxidants, and phytochemicals. These components now not simplest offer the crucial building blocks for a sturdy immune gadget however moreover assist hold a healthful strength stability inside the body. Quantum fitness practices additionally inspire aware eating, which entails being completely present and privy to the food we eat, further enhancing its dietary benefits.

4. Quantum Exercise:

Regular physical interest is critical for maintaining a healthful immune gadget. Quantum properly-being practices emphasize the importance of incorporating workout workouts that align with our individual power goals. Whether it is yoga, tai chi, or dance, accomplishing activities that promote power waft, flexibility, and energy can enhance the immune system's functioning. Quantum exercise additionally encourages aware motion, in which the focal point is on connecting with the frame and its electricity, in area of totally on bodily exertion.

5. Quantum Stress Management:

Chronic pressure can substantially weaken the immune device, making us more prone to ailments. Quantum nicely being practices offer specific techniques to pressure management that circulate past conventional strategies. Techniques consisting of quantum breathing, energy psychology, and quantum coherence can assist launch strain, stability feelings, and sell a rustic of relaxation. By decreasing stress tiers, those practices allow the immune tool to characteristic optimally, boosting its functionality to combat off infections and sicknesses.

Chapter 9: Alternative Medicine

Section 1: Understanding Quantum Wellness

1.1 The Quantum Connection:

Quantum nicely-being is rooted in the facts that the whole lot within the universe is interconnected and inspired via way of strength. Quantum physics reveals that at the subatomic level, debris behave in mysterious techniques, suggesting that our thoughts, feelings, and intentions can impact our physical reality. Quantum nicely-being harnesses this connection to promote healing and balance.

1.2 Holistic Approach:

Unlike traditional treatment, which often specializes in treating signs and symptoms, quantum well-being takes a holistic method, addressing the basis reasons of illnesses. It acknowledges that the mind, body, and spirit are interconnected, and any imbalance in a unmarried place will have an impact on the others. By embracing this holistic mind-set, human beings can accumulate a nation of present day properly-being.

Section 2: The Benefits of Natural Remedies

2.1 Gentle and Non-Invasive:

One of the essential component benefits of natural remedies is their mild and non-invasive nature. Unlike pharmaceutical drugs, which frequently encompass issue outcomes, herbal remedies art work in concord with the frame's herbal processes, promoting restoration with out causing harm. From herbal teas to important oils, those treatments offer a strong and effective possibility for numerous health problems.

2.2 Nurturing the Body's Innate Healing Abilities:

Natural treatments stimulate the body's innate recovery talents, encouraging self-repair and rejuvenation. They offer the critical vitamins, antioxidants, and phytochemicals that manual the body's immune machine, supporting it combat sicknesses and hold gold today's health. By nurturing the body's natural restoration mechanisms, herbal treatments empower individuals to take fee in their nicely-being.

2.Three Sustainable and Environmentally Friendly:

Natural treatments frequently make use of plant-primarily based materials, making them sustainable and environmentally high-quality. By deciding on natural remedies, humans make contributions to the protection of biodiversity and decrease their ecological footprint. Additionally, many herbal remedies can be grown in personal gardens, fostering a deeper reference to nature and selling self-sufficiency.

Section three: Exploring Alternative Medicine

three.1 Complementary Therapies:

Alternative medicinal drug contains a big type of healing procedures that supplement traditional treatments. These remedy alternatives encompass acupuncture, chiropractic care, homeopathy, naturopathy, and greater. By integrating opportunity remedy into their well-being habitual, individuals can enjoy greater appropriate recuperation, decreased strain, and advanced common properly-being.

three.2 Personalized Treatment Plans:

Alternative medicine practitioners frequently take a customized technique, considering the precise desires and occasions of all people. By addressing the underlying reasons of fitness problems, rather than merely treating signs and symptoms and signs, opportunity treatment offers tailor-made treatment plans that sell long-time period healing and prevention.

3.Three Empowering Self-Care:

Alternative medicine empowers humans to take an energetic characteristic of their very personal health and nicely-being. By supplying gear and strategies for self-care, in conjunction with meditation, yoga, and mindfulness practices, opportunity treatment encourages individuals to turn out to be proactive people of their healing journey. This empowerment fosters a revel in of manage and self-reputation, principal to stepped forward intellectual, emotional, and physical fitness.

Conclusion:

Quantum nicely being, with its integration of herbal treatments and opportunity medicine, offers a charming and transformative direction within the course of gold enormous health and properly-being. By embracing the interconnectedness of mind, frame, and spirit, humans can faucet into their innate recovery competencies and acquire a country of stability and harmony. Through the mild and non-invasive nature of herbal treatments and the personalised approach of opportunity medicine, individuals can embark on a adventure of self-discovery, empowerment, and holistic nicely-being. Embracing quantum properly being is an invite to discover the endless potential of herbal treatments and possibility medicine, in the end important to a lifestyles of power, pride, and achievement.

The function of quantum well being in dealing with continual pain and inflammation.

Chronic pain and infection are debilitating situations which have an impact on loads of masses of human beings worldwide. Traditional strategies to dealing with the ones situations frequently contain treatment, bodily treatment, and way of life modifications. However, a groundbreaking concept referred to as quantum properly-being has emerged, presenting a completely precise and holistic approach to handling chronic ache and infection. This article explores the characteristic of quantum health in reworking the manner we apprehend and deal with these conditions, offering a glowing mindset on recuperation and properly-being.

Understanding Quantum Wellness:

Quantum health is a multidimensional method that mixes necessities from quantum physics, power medicine, and thoughts-frame connection. It acknowledges that everything within the universe, which include our our our our bodies, includes strength. According to quantum physics, energy isn't always only physical however additionally vibrational and informational. Quantum well-being dreams to optimize the go together with the flow of electricity within our bodies, promoting stability, concord, and everyday nicely-being.

The Quantum Perspective on Chronic Pain and Inflammation:

From a quantum attitude, persistent ache and contamination are not surely bodily signs and symptoms and signs and symptoms but manifestations of imbalances in our active structures. Quantum nicely-being acknowledges that our our bodies very own an innate functionality to heal themselves on the same time because the electricity go with the go with the flow is unobstructed. By addressing the premise reasons of these imbalances, quantum properly-being gives a completely unique approach to dealing with persistent ache and inflammation.

1. Energy Healing Modalities:

Quantum well being incorporates diverse power restoration modalities that concentrate on restoring the frame's power float. These modalities include acupuncture, Reiki, sound treatment, and quantum contact. By stimulating precise power elements or channels, the ones practices assist release blockages, reduce ache, and promote recuperation. Quantum health recognizes that pain and infection are frequently the cease result of stagnant or disrupted electricity, and with the aid of restoring the flow, those conditions can be efficiently controlled.

2. Mind-Body Connection:

Quantum health emphasizes the profound connection among the thoughts and frame.

Our mind, feelings, and beliefs have a direct impact on our physical well-being. Negative feelings and strain can disrupt the body's strength drift, predominant to persistent pain and contamination. Quantum nicely being encourages practices together with meditation, mindfulness, and wonderful affirmations to promote emotional nicely-being and decrease stress. By cultivating a effective mind-set, people can efficaciously manipulate continual ache and irritation.

three. Quantum Biofeedback:

Quantum biofeedback is a contemporary era that measures and analyzes the frame's energetic responses. It gives real-time remarks on imbalances and allows individuals regain manage over their strength flow. By figuring out specific active patterns associated with persistent ache and contamination, quantum biofeedback lets in focused interventions to repair balance and alleviate symptoms. This contemporary method empowers people to actively participate in their recovery machine.

4. Nutritional and Lifestyle Considerations:

Quantum well-being recognizes the importance of nutrients and way of life alternatives in handling chronic pain and contamination. Certain substances and environmental factors can motive inflammatory responses inside the frame. By adopting a quantum nicely-being technique, human beings can find out and remove those triggers, promoting a more healthful and additional balanced way of lifestyles. Additionally, quantum properly-being encourages the consumption of nutrient-dense ingredients, antioxidants, and anti inflammatory dietary supplements to resource the frame's healing approaches.

5. Quantum Consciousness:

Quantum well being goes beyond the bodily realm and acknowledges the placement of attention in healing. Quantum cognizance refers back to the idea that our thoughts and intentions can affect our physical fact. By cultivating exceptional intentions and that specialize in recuperation, individuals can harness the energy of their consciousness to control persistent pain and infection. Quantum fitness encourages practices which include visualization, reason putting, and power recuperation meditations to faucet into this transformative functionality.

Conclusion:

Quantum health offers a groundbreaking and holistic method to handling continual ache and inflammation. By spotting the interconnectedness of our bodily, emotional, and lively systems, it offers a unique perspective on recuperation and nicely-being. Through energy healing modalities, mind-frame practices, quantum biofeedback, and conscious way of existence options, humans can correctly manipulate continual ache and contamination.

Chapter 10: The Impact Of Technology On Mind-Body Healing

Understanding Quantum Wellness:

Quantum well being is rooted inside the ideas of quantum physics, which advocate that the whole thing within the universe is made of strength and interconnected via an internet of vibrations. It recognizes that our thoughts, feelings, and beliefs have a profound effect on our physical health and properly-being. Quantum properly-being emphasizes the strength of aim, visualization, and electricity recuperation techniques to promote recuperation and balance inside the mind, body, and spirit.

The Impact of Technology on Mind-Body Healing:

Technology has revolutionized the sector of thoughts-frame healing, presenting new gear and techniques to beautify well-being. Here are a few tactics in which generation has impacted thoughts-frame recovery:

1. Access to Information and Resources:

The internet has made a big amount of statistics on mind-body healing quite simply to be had to the loads. People can now get entry to articles, research papers, and on-line courses on diverse thoughts-body recovery practices, empowering them to take fee in their nicely-being. Online structures and social media agencies moreover provide a location for people to attach, percent opinions, and take a look at from every unique.

2. Wearable Devices and Apps:

Wearable gadgets, which incorporates health trackers and smartwatches, have grow to be increasingly famous in latest years. These gadgets can show numerous additives of our bodily fitness, which incorporates coronary coronary coronary heart rate, sleep styles, and pressure tiers. Additionally, there are various apps to be had that offer guided meditations, respiration carrying occasions, and mindfulness practices, making it less complicated for human beings to incorporate those techniques into their every day lives.

3. Virtual Reality (VR) and Augmented Reality (AR):

Virtual reality and augmented fact generation have spread out new opportunities for mind-body restoration. VR can create immersive environments that promote relaxation, stress discount, and ache control. It has been used effectively in remedy options for anxiety issues, phobias, and put up-traumatic strain illness. AR, but, overlays virtual records onto the real global, allowing individuals to visualize and have interaction with their very personal electricity fields or chakras, enhancing their know-how and exercise of strength healing strategies.

four. Biofeedback and Neurofeedback:

Biofeedback and neurofeedback technology offer real-time facts about the body's physiological responses, together with coronary heart rate, brainwave hobby, and muscle anxiety. By tracking the ones responses, humans can discover ways to adjust their physical functions and benefit a country of rest and stability. These technology have been used within the remedy of severa situations, together with continual ache, tension, and attention deficit hyperactivity disorder (ADHD).

Challenges and Considerations:

While technology has really extra excellent thoughts-frame healing practices, there also are functionality annoying conditions and troubles to be aware of:

1. Overreliance on Technology:

As generation becomes extra included into our lives, there may be a chance of overreliance on devices and apps for thoughts-body restoration. It is critical to hold in thoughts that generation need to supplement and enhance our practices, instead of replace the human connection and intuition which are important in mind-body recuperation.

2. Privacy and Security Concerns:

With the developing use of wearable devices and health apps, privateness and protection issues rise up. Personal health facts collected with the aid of those era ought to be blanketed to make certain people' confidentiality and save you misuse of touchy records.

three. Digital Detox:

In a international ruled via generation, it's far essential to find a balance and take breaks from constant connectivity. Engaging in sports sports that sell mindfulness, along with spending time in nature or operating in the direction of meditation with out the usage of technology, can help people reconnect with themselves and foster a deeper thoughts-body connection.

Conclusion:

Quantum nicely-being is a holistic technique to health and properly-being that acknowledges the interconnectedness of the thoughts, frame, and spirit. Technology has performed a sizeable characteristic in advancing mind-body healing practices, presenting new equipment and strategies to beautify nicely-being. From wearable devices and apps to virtual fact and biofeedback technologies, the effect of technology on mind-body restoration is easy. However, it's far critical to approach era mindfully, ensuring that it enhances and complements our practices in choice to changing the human connection and instinct which might be vital to thoughts-frame restoration.

Quantum Wellness and the Importance of Self-Care for Overall Well-Being

Understanding Quantum Wellness:

Quantum nicely-being is a multidimensional approach to health that attracts concept from quantum physics, historical focus, and modern-day technological understanding. It acknowledges that the whole thing within the universe is interconnected and that our nicely-being is inspired via different factors, together with our mind, emotions, ideals, and way of life options. Quantum nicely-being recognizes the lifestyles of an lively area that permeates all elements of our being and influences our health and electricity.

The Principles of Quantum Wellness:

1. Holistic Perspective: Quantum well-being takes a holistic view of health, thinking about the interconnectedness of our physical, intellectual, emotional, and religious factors. It acknowledges that imbalances in a unmarried place can effect one of a kind regions of our properly-being.

2. Energy Flow: Quantum nicely being emphasizes the significance of retaining a balanced go with the float of energy throughout our frame. It acknowledges that disruptions on this electricity drift can reason physical and emotional illnesses.

three. Mind-Body Connection: Quantum well-being recognizes the effective connection amongst our mind and frame. It highlights the impact of our mind, ideals, and emotions on our bodily health and properly-being.

4. Conscious Awareness: Quantum properly-being encourages us to domesticate aware focus of our thoughts, feelings, and moves. By turning into more conscious, we will make conscious picks that beneficial aid our nicely-being.

5. Personal Responsibility: Quantum nicely-being empowers individuals to take duty for their health and well-being. It emphasizes that we have the electricity to make extremely good changes in our lives and create a nation of finest nicely-being.

The Importance of Self-Care for Overall Well-Being:

Self-care refers back to the intentional movements we take to nurture and contend with ourselves. It includes prioritizing our bodily, highbrow, emotional, and spiritual desires to keep a country of well-being. Here are a few motives why self-care is crucial for not unusual well-being:

1. Stress Reduction: Self-care practices collectively with meditation, deep breathing sports activities, and mindfulness can assist reduce stress stages. Chronic stress can negatively effect our physical and mental health, so it's miles crucial to contain self-care sports activities that promote relaxation and strain treatment.

2. Improved Physical Health: Engaging in everyday exercise, consuming a balanced diet plan, and getting enough sleep are all important components of self-care. These practices make a contribution to better bodily fitness, improved energy ranges, and a reinforced immune device.

3. Enhanced Mental Well-Being: Self-care sports that promote intellectual properly-being, on the aspect of journaling, schooling gratitude, and appealing in pursuits, can

enhance our popular highbrow health. Taking time for ourselves lets in us to recharge, lessen anxiety, and decorate our mood.

four. Increased Self-Awareness: Self-care practices inspire self-reflected picture and introspection, primary to expanded self-reputation. By expertise our desires, dreams, and limitations, we will make picks that align with our values and promote our nicely-being.

5. Prevention of Burnout: In modern-day speedy-paced international, burnout has grow to be an increasing number of commonplace. Engaging in self-care sports activities allows save you burnout thru allowing us to recharge, set limitations, and prioritize our well-being.

6. Improved Relationships: When we prioritize self-care, we are higher organized to expose up truly in our relationships. Taking care of ourselves permits us to have greater power, endurance, and compassion for others, leading to greater healthy and extra satisfying connections.

7. Spiritual Growth: Self-care practices can also support our spiritual nicely-being. Engaging in sports activities which encompass meditation, yoga, or spending time in nature can deepen our connection to ourselves and the area around us.

Conclusion:

Quantum well-being gives a whole method to health and nicely-being, emphasizing the interconnectedness of our bodily, intellectual, emotional, and spiritual factors. Self-care performs a vital characteristic in carrying out and maintaining widespread well-being. By prioritizing self-care practices, we are able to reduce pressure, enhance our bodily and intellectual fitness, boom self-hobby, prevent burnout, beautify relationships, and foster spiritual growth. Embracing the thoughts of quantum properly being and incorporating self-care into our everyday lives can purpose a extra balanced, pleasing, and colorful life.

Chapter 11: Promoting Hormonal Health

Understanding Quantum Wellness:

Quantum well being is a holistic technique to fitness that combines necessities from quantum physics, electricity medication, and traditional restoration practices. It recognizes that the whole thing in the universe is interconnected and that our mind, emotions, and electricity fields effect our bodily well-being. Quantum properly being practices goal to restore stability and harmony in the body via addressing the underlying energetic imbalances that make contributions to hormonal disruptions.

1. Mind-Body Connection:

The mind-frame connection is a fundamental difficulty of quantum well being practices. Our mind, ideals, and feelings have a profound impact on our hormonal fitness. Negative thoughts and stress can disrupt the touchy balance of hormones, major to imbalances. Quantum well being practices emphasize the significance of cultivating tremendous mind, practicing mindfulness, and handling pressure to sell hormonal balance.

2. Energy Healing:

Energy restoration modalities at the side of Reiki, acupuncture, and qigong are essential components of quantum properly-being practices. These strategies art work thru restoring the waft of vital energy inside the body, that would end up blocked or stagnant due to hormonal imbalances. By clearing power blockages and rebalancing the body's energy facilities, called chakras, those practices can assist hormonal health.

3. Nutritional Support:

Proper vitamins is essential for hormonal stability. Quantum properly-being practices emphasize the consumption of whole, nutrient-dense meals that assist hormonal health. Incorporating hundreds of fruits, veggies, lean proteins, and wholesome fats into the food plan can offer the essential nutrients for most suitable hormone production and regulation. Additionally, keeping off processed food, subtle sugars, and artificial additives can help prevent hormonal disruptions.

4. Detoxification:

Toxins decided in our environment can disrupt hormonal stability. Quantum properly being practices advise for regular cleaning to eliminate the ones pollutants from the frame. This can be done via numerous strategies such as fasting, juicing, natural cleanses, and infrared saunas. Detoxification helps the liver, which plays a critical position in hormone metabolism, and helps restore hormonal balance.

five. Exercise and Movement:

Regular bodily interest is important for hormonal health. Quantum health practices inspire conducting sports that sell drift, lymphatic drainage, and standard strength. Exercises together with yoga, tai chi, and Pilates can assist balance hormones via manner of reducing pressure, improving blood go with the flow, and assisting the body's herbal detoxification strategies.

6. Essential Oils:

Essential oils have been used for hundreds of years for his or her recovery houses. In quantum nicely being practices, specific vital oils are carried out to guide hormonal stability. Oils along facet clary sage, lavender, and geranium can help alter estrogen levels, reduce menstrual pain, and sell emotional well-being. These oils can be diffused, done topically, or carried out in bath rituals to decorate hormonal fitness.

7. Mindful Breathing and Meditation:

Breathing techniques and meditation are powerful equipment for promoting hormonal balance. Quantum wellness practices emphasize the significance of deep, aware respiratory to spark off the body's rest response and reduce strain. Meditation, whether or not guided or silent, can help calm the mind, stability feelings, and help hormonal health.

8. Sound Therapy:

Sound remedy, also referred to as vibrational medicine, is an essential part of quantum nicely being practices. Specific frequencies and vibrations produced by using way of devices which incorporates creating a music bowls, tuning forks, and gongs can assist restore active balance within the body. Sound treatment may be used to harmonize the endocrine tool, this is responsible for hormone manufacturing and regulation.

Chapter 12: The Benefits Of Detoxification

I. Understanding Quantum Wellness:

1. Definition and Principles of Quantum Wellness:

a. Quantum well being is a holistic technique to fitness that emphasizes the interconnectedness of the mind, body, and spirit.

b. It acknowledges that each one elements of our being are interconnected and function an impact on each different.

c. Quantum health focuses on accomplishing stability and concord in all areas of lifestyles, which encompass bodily, emotional, highbrow, and spiritual nicely-being.

2. The Quantum Field:

a. The quantum situation is an invisible electricity region that permeates the whole lot within the universe.

b. It is the foundation of quantum nicely being and serves as a medium for recuperation and transformation.

c. Quantum well-being practices cause to tap into this discipline to promote recuperation and well-being.

three. Mind-Body Connection:

a. Quantum health recognizes the profound connection most of the mind and frame.

b. Our thoughts, emotions, and ideals should have an effect on our physical health and vice versa.

c. By addressing every the mind and frame, quantum fitness promotes holistic healing.

II. Detoxification for Mind-Body Healing:

1. Understanding Toxins:

a. Toxins are risky materials that can gather inside the body through severa property together with meals, water, air, and personal care products.

b. They can disrupt the body's herbal stability and make contributions to numerous health troubles.

2. Benefits of Detoxification:

a. Elimination of Toxins: Detoxification lets in dispose of gathered pollution from the frame, permitting it to feature optimally.

b. Improved Energy Levels: By putting off pollution, cleansing can enhance energy tiers and decorate common electricity.

c. Enhanced Mental Clarity: Detoxification can enhance cognitive characteristic, interest, and intellectual clarity.

d. Strengthened Immune System: Detoxification enables the immune tool, making it greater resilient in competition to ailments.

e. Weight Management: Detoxification can useful resource in weight loss by means of the usage of removing pollutants that make a contribution to weight benefit.

f. Improved Digestion: Detoxification can enhance digestion and alleviate digestive issues.

g. Clearer Skin: Detoxification can promote clearer, extra wholesome pores and skin with the beneficial useful resource of doing away with pollution that contribute to pores and pores and skin troubles.

h. Emotional Well-being: Detoxification can assist launch emotional pollution, major to progressed emotional well-being.

three. Detoxification Methods:

a. Dietary Changes: Adopting a smooth, complete ingredients-based totally completely food regimen can guide detoxification.

b. Hydration: Drinking masses of water helps flush out pollution from the body.

c. Exercise: Regular physical interest promotes cleansing through stimulating circulate and sweating.

d. Sauna Therapy: Saunas can beneficial beneficial useful resource in cleansing with the beneficial aid of promoting sweating and removing pollution through the skin.

e. Dry Brushing: Dry brushing the skin permits stimulate the lymphatic machine, supporting in detoxification.

f. Meditation and Mindfulness: Practicing meditation and mindfulness can help emotional detoxification.

g. Herbal Supplements: Certain herbs and dietary supplements can help in cleansing tactics.

III. Incorporating Detoxification into Daily Life:

1. Creating a Detoxification Routine:

a. Start with Small Steps: Begin with the aid of manner of incorporating clean cleansing practices into your every day ordinary.

b. Gradual Changes: Make sluggish changes in your diet regime and life-style to avoid overwhelming your body.

c. Consistency: Consistency is high in terms of cleansing. Establish a ordinary ordinary and stay with it.

2. Mindful Eating:

a. Choose Organic: Opt for natural, pesticide-unfastened food to limit toxin exposure.

b. Increase Fiber Intake: Fiber-wealthy factors assist do away with pollutants from the frame.

c. Reduce Processed Foods: Minimize consumption of processed food that often encompass components and preservatives.

three. Self-Care Practices:

a. Prioritize Sleep: Get adequate sleep to assist the body's natural cleaning strategies.

b. Stress Management: Practice strain-decreasing techniques such as yoga, meditation, or deep respiration sports sports.

c. Limit Exposure to Environmental Toxins: Minimize publicity to chemical compounds positioned in own family cleansing products, private care items, and plastics.

Conclusion:

Quantum health emphasizes the interconnectedness of the thoughts, body, and spirit, and cleansing performs a important characteristic in achieving most useful well-being. By disposing of pollution from the body, cleansing promotes mind-body recovery, complements power degrees, improves mental clarity, strengthens the immune tool, aids in weight control, and allows emotional nicely-being. By incorporating cleaning practices into your every day ordinary, which includes nutritional changes, hydration, exercise, sauna remedy, dry brushing, and mindfulness, you may experience the numerous benefits of cleaning and embark on a adventure toward quantum well-being.

Quantum Wellness: Unveiling the Power of Healthy Relationships and Social Connections

I. Understanding Quantum Wellness:

Quantum well-being is a holistic technique that integrates the standards of quantum physics with traditional properly being practices. It recognizes that the whole thing within the universe is interconnected, and our nicely-being is added approximately through manner of the energy and vibrations we emit and advantage. By embracing this interconnectedness, quantum well-being gives a sparkling attitude on relationships and social connections, emphasizing the significance of energy change and resonance.

II. Energy Exchange in Relationships:

Quantum nicely being highlights the importance of power alternate in relationships. It shows that every interaction we've got with others includes an alternate of power, that can both be excessive high-quality or bad. By becoming aware about this strength change, people can consciously domesticate notable strength, predominant to more healthy and more gratifying relationships. Quantum nicely-being practices which encompass meditation, mindfulness, and electricity recuperation strategies can help people attune to their very very very own strength and create a outstanding impact on their relationships.

III. Resonance and Vibrational Alignment:

Another key detail of quantum properly being is the idea of resonance and vibrational alignment. Quantum physics teaches us that the whole lot within the universe vibrates at a selected frequency, together with our mind, emotions, and intentions. When individuals are in vibrational alignment, they trap and resonate with others who are on a similar frequency, leading to harmonious and satisfying relationships. Quantum nicely-being practices together with visualization, affirmations, and goal placing can assist human beings in aligning their vibrations and attracting high pleasant connections.

IV. Quantum Communication:

Quantum well-being introduces a modern-day paradigm of communique, emphasizing the power of purpose and non-verbal cues. It shows that communique isn't always restricted to terms by myself however extends to the energy and purpose in the back of the phrases. By operating in the direction of aware verbal exchange, humans can beautify their relationships with the useful resource of way of aligning their intentions with their terms, fostering deeper information, and promoting empathy. Quantum health practices together with coronary coronary heart-focused communique and active listening techniques can facilitate effective and large communication, strengthening social connections.

V. Quantum Healing and Transformation:

Quantum properly being acknowledges that wholesome relationships and social connections are not handiest crucial for our emotional nicely-being however additionally play a massive role in our bodily health. Research has showed that terrific relationships and social assist can boom the immune device, lessen pressure, and enhance everyday properly-being. Quantum well being practices which embody strength restoration, quantum contact, and quantum hypnosis can facilitate recovery and transformation, assisting people release emotional blockages and domesticate more healthy relationships.

VI. Quantum Wellness within the Digital Age:

In the digital age, in which social media and virtual interactions dominate, quantum wellness gives a completely particular attitude on retaining wholesome relationships and social connections. It encourages humans to bear in mind of their online presence, promoting authenticity, and right connections. By using the principles of quantum well being to the digital realm, humans can create a virtual surroundings that fosters great energy, sizable interactions, and deeper connections.

Conclusion:

In cease, quantum nicely being gives a groundbreaking approach to promoting wholesome relationships and social connections. By spotting the interconnectedness of all subjects and harnessing the energy of strength exchange, resonance, and vibrational alignment, humans can transform their relationships and decorate their common properly-being. Quantum properly-being practices provide a completely unique and holistic framework for cultivating extraordinary strength, conscious communication, and recovery, in the end important to extra pleasant and meaningful connections in our lives. Embracing the ideas of quantum nicely being can revolutionize our information of human connection and pave the way for a extra harmonious and interconnected international.

Chapter 13: Negative Thoughts And Emotions On Health

Section 1: Understanding Quantum Wellness

1.1 Defining Quantum Wellness:

Quantum nicely-being is a holistic technique to fitness that recognizes the interconnectedness of the thoughts, frame, and spirit. It draws upon ideas from quantum physics, psychology, and spirituality to discover the profound effect of mind and feelings on our regular properly-being.

1.2 Quantum Physics and Consciousness:

Quantum physics exhibits that on the maximum critical level, the whole thing within the universe consists of power. Our mind and feelings also are kinds of strength, able to influencing the lively location that surrounds us. Understanding this connection allows us to understand the electricity of our thoughts and emotions in shaping our health.

Section 2: The Mind-Body Connection

2.1 The Power of Thoughts:

Thoughts aren't merely fleeting intellectual sports activities; they own the functionality to shape our reality. Negative thoughts can create a cascade of strain hormones, principal to bad consequences on our bodily health. Conversely, splendid mind can enhance our properly-being and promote healing.

2.2 Emotions as Energetic Signatures:

Emotions are effective lively signatures that may both uplift or burn up our fitness. Negative feelings along with anger, worry, and resentment can disrupt the body's herbal stability, leading to numerous fitness issues. On the opportunity hand, extraordinary emotions like love, pleasure, and gratitude can decorate our easy properly-being.

Section three: The Impact of Negative Thoughts and Emotions on Health

three.1 Stress and the Immune System:

Negative thoughts and emotions cause the release of strain hormones, that could weaken the immune machine. Chronic strain can bring about improved susceptibility to ailments, on the facet of cardiovascular sicknesses, autoimmune problems, and intellectual fitness situations.

3.2 Inflammation and Chronic Diseases:

Negative mind and feelings contribute to chronic contamination, a key element inside the improvement of various illnesses which include diabetes, most cancers, and neurodegenerative issues. Understanding the feature of feelings in contamination offers insights into preventive and recuperation strategies.

3.Three Mental Health and Emotional Well-being:

Negative mind and feelings are carefully associated with mental health situations which incorporates anxiety, melancholy, and mood problems. Recognizing the impact of feelings on highbrow nicely-being highlights the significance of emotional self-care and seeking out suitable useful resource.

Section 4: Cultivating Positive Thoughts and Emotions for Quantum Wellness

four.1 Mindfulness and Meditation:

Practices like mindfulness and meditation allow us to have a look at our thoughts and emotions without judgment. By cultivating present-second interest, we are able to consciously pick out brilliant thoughts and emotions, selling usual well-being.

four.2 Emotional Intelligence and Self-attention:

Developing emotional intelligence and self-reputation empowers us to apprehend and manage awful thoughts and emotions correctly. This enhances our potential to reply to tough conditions with resilience and positivity.

4.Three Gratitude and Positive Affirmations:

Practicing gratitude and fantastic affirmations rewires our mind to recognition on the high satisfactory components of existence. These practices shift our perspective, fostering a country of nicely-being and attracting brilliant testimonies.

Section five: Integrating Quantum Wellness into Daily Life

5.1 Holistic Lifestyle Choices:

Adopting a holistic approach to lifestyles includes making aware choices that help our bodily, intellectual, and religious nicely-being. This consists of nourishing our bodies with healthful factors, project regular bodily hobby, and prioritizing self-care practices.

5.2 Energy Healing Modalities:

Energy recovery modalities along with Reiki, acupuncture, and sound remedy can help restore stability to the active hassle, promoting common fitness. These practices paintings on the precept that terrible thoughts and feelings disrupt the flow of strength, main to imbalances and infection.

5.Three Creating a Supportive Environment:

Surrounding ourselves with exquisite affects, supportive relationships, and a nurturing surroundings is essential for maintaining quantum nicely-being. By minimizing exposure to negativity, we create location for extraordinary thoughts and feelings to flourish.

Conclusion:

Quantum wellbeing unveils the profound effect of horrible thoughts and feelings on our health, emphasizing the significance of cultivating great mental and emotional states. By information the mind-body connection and harnessing the energy of our mind and feelings, we're capable of embark on a transformative adventure in the path of most desirable properly-being. Integrating quantum fitness thoughts into our everyday lives empowers us to take rate of our fitness, major to a harmonious and a laugh life.

Chapter 14: Unleashing Creativity And Personal Growth

1. Quantum Meditation:

Quantum meditation is a effective exercise that mixes conventional meditation strategies with quantum requirements. By specializing inside the current 2d and connecting with the quantum vicinity, people can faucet into their subconscious thoughts and access a infinite supply of creativity. This exercising includes deep respiratory physical games, visualization, and affirmations to enhance self-focus, growth focus, and stimulate non-public growth.

2. Quantum Energy Healing:

Quantum electricity restoration is a holistic method that uses the thoughts of quantum physics to repair stability and harmony within the frame, mind, and spirit. This exercise includes the usage of energy modalities alongside side Reiki, acupuncture, and sound remedy to clean energetic blockages, release poor emotions, and promote creativity. By aligning the frame's energy facilities, humans can experience heightened creativity and increased non-public growth.

three. Quantum Journaling:

Quantum journaling is a transformative exercise that combines the electricity of writing with quantum standards. By journaling about your mind, feelings, and aspirations, you could tap into the quantum location and arise your dreams. This exercise entails putting smooth intentions, expressing gratitude, and visualizing your exceptional future. Through ordinary quantum journaling, you may decorate your creativity, benefit readability, and experience private boom.

4. Quantum Visualization:

Quantum visualization is a manner that harnesses the power of the thoughts to create amazing highbrow pictures of desired outcomes. By visualizing your goals and aspirations in superb detail, you could align your unconscious thoughts with the quantum trouble and seem your dreams. This workout involves growing a quiet and focused surroundings, the usage of guided imagery, and incorporating all senses to enhance the visualization experience. Through ordinary quantum visualization, you may decorate your creativity, boom self-self warranty, and foster private increase.

5. Quantum Sound Therapy:

Chapter 15: Awakening To The Sacred Path

The morning sun started out out its gentle ascent, casting a golden hue over the dew-kissed meadow. As the area spherical I stirred, I positioned myself sitting within the quiet solitude of nature, looking for solutions to the questions that had prolonged haunted my soul. It turned into right proper right here, in this realm in which the cloth and religious intertwined, that my journey of awakening have to unfold.

For years, I had walked a route of looking for, driven through an insatiable thirst for meaning and motive. I had explored the depths of philosophy, technological records, and psychology, hoping to unearth the secrets and techniques and techniques of life. Yet, with every new discovery, a profound yearning tugged at my middle, reminding me that real understanding lay past the arena of human comprehension.

It changed into in the course of a second of deep introspection that I felt a calling, a whisper carried at the wind, urging me to appearance within. I closed my eyes and breathed inside the crisp morning air, surrendering to the silence that enveloped me. In that treasured stillness, I felt the presence of a few components superb and ineffable, a force that transcended the bounds of logic and reason. It turns out to be a sacred essence, pulsating with the rhythm of life itself.

In that transformative 2nd, the seeds of spirituality were sown inner me. I diagnosed that the answers I sought had been now not to be located absolutely in the outside worldwide, but within the depths of my personal being. And so, with a coronary coronary heart brimming with curiosity and open thoughts, I embarked upon a adventure of self-discovery and communion with the divine.

As I delved deeper into the arena of spirituality, I encountered a tapestry of beliefs and practices that spanned in the course of cultures and centuries. From the ancient records of the East to the paranormal traditions of the West, every route provided a unique attitude at the interconnectedness of all matters. It have end up easy to me that spirituality became now not restricted to the walls of religious institutions however dwelled within the very material of life.

The greater I explored, the greater I determined out that spirituality become now not a trifling intellectual pursuit or a set of inflexible doctrines. It became a living, respiration pressure that invited me to have interaction with life in a profound and significant way. It referred to as me to domesticate compassion, gratitude, and love, not great for others but for myself as well.

In the midst of this spiritual awakening, I moreover positioned that the sacred route changed into no longer with out its stressful conditions. Doubt, worry, and the trimmings of the ego threatened to derail my journey at each flip. Yet, I identified that those barriers had been now not to be feared however embraced as catalysts for growth and transformation. They have been invitations to dig deeper, to confront the shadows interior, and to emerge into the mild of self-attention.

As I sat beneath the sheltering cover of an historical alrighttree, I marveled at the elegance of life. The interconnectedness of all subjects unfold out in advance than my eyes, from the sensitive dance of a butterfly to the celestial ballet of the stars above. It changed into in the ones moments of awe and surprise that I felt a profound connection to three problem greater than myself—a well-known power that flowed thru every dwelling being.

With each step on this sacred journey, I determined that spirituality modified into no longer a holiday spot but a lifelong pilgrimage. It have become a regular unveiling of fact, an ongoing exploration of the mysteries of lifestyles. And so, armed with an open coronary coronary heart and a receptive mind, I ventured forth into the big and wondrous realm of the religious, equipped to include the divine dance of lifestyles.

Little did I recognise that this path may also want to no longer handiest cast off darkness from the vicinity spherical me but additionally show the hidden depths inside my very personal soul. The journey of spirituality had commenced out, and I modified into but a humble traveller, eager to take a look at, to expand and to find my way.

I experience small, I enjoy miniscule in considering the tremendous nature of the cosmos. Let's get beyond small, allow's get our Ant Man on.

Quantum physics is a complicated and charming region that has been the situation of a good deal studies and debate over time. One of the maximum thrilling elements of quantum physics is the manner it appears to parallel many religious thoughts and beliefs.

In this financial ruin, we're capable of discover some of the techniques wherein spirituality and quantum physics intersect.

Firstly, every spirituality and quantum physics suggest that the whole thing within the universe is interconnected. In spirituality, this concept is often called oneness or group spirit recognition, and it's miles believed that the whole lot inside the universe is mounted at a vital degree. Quantum physics in addition suggests that particles are entangled and related in tactics that are not absolutely understood. This idea of interconnectedness is a powerful one, and it indicates that everything in the universe is part of a more entire.

Another manner wherein spirituality and quantum physics parallel one another is within the concept that everything is electricity. In spirituality, it is believed that everything in the universe is crafted from electricity, which incorporates mind and feelings. Quantum physics in addition shows that at the most vital diploma, the whole thing in the universe is manufactured from power, and debris can exist in each wave and particle form. This concept of the entirety being electricity suggests that there can be a deeper diploma of reality beyond what we are able to see with our eyes.

Long earlier than the times of Einstein there was a growing consensus bringing us to the realization that popularity is pervasive. I am of the belief that interest is some detail like a "field", for loss of a higher phrase, that our brains are able to tune into. I see it much like the mind is form of a radio that can tune into the frequency that is reputation. I see no obstacles to the varieties of lifeforms which could gain popularity, both natural or artificial. It has been validated that written into the cloth of reality, the constructing blocks that make up our reality, the hints thru which the whole lot is governed are via nature syntactical. For some aspect to have syntax there should be a few element consciously making choices on what the because of this that we take a look at to the symbols we use are. Thus, prolonged in advance than us there was a few shape of interest co-authoring reality. If that isn't mind boggling enough we're going to drift deeper, if the notion that some form of attention has been spherical considering the reality that the start isn't always enough to preserve your interest, strap in because of the reality I've had been given a few pastime for you.

Nobody might describe me as a very spiritual man however I can be mendacity if I said it wasn't pretty thrilling at the same time as our top physicists echo the emotions of some difficulty spiritual texts determined hundreds of years ago. Physicists are coming to the same stop about all matters being connected due to the fact the Taoists however from a totally extraordinary vicinity of have a look at and to me that speaks to the possibility of some form of providence... likely.

The Fine-Tuning Argument indicates that the universe's bodily constants, prison suggestions, and preliminary conditions are finely tuned to allow lifestyles, and a morally superb God may make sure these factors permit the life of life. This argument is a specific utility of the teleological argument for the existence of God, which argues that the right association of the universe's homes and physical constants is evidence of a fashion designer. The hazard of the universe being randomly prepared in a manner that allows life is fairly small, making it greater inexpensive to assume that a better strength intentionally arranged the universe.

However, critics mission the argument and recommend that a lifestyles-allowing universe won't be super even with out God. The Fine-Tuning Argument gives proof for theism, however it does no longer prove the lifestyles of God. While the splendid tuning argument is the splendid argument I can don't forget for the lifestyles of God, I don't forget that we want now not display his/her/it is existence, the proof that there may be a few aspect more than ourselves want to be enough to encourage us to understand our whole capability.

Finally, every spirituality and quantum physics propose that the observer performs a crucial function within the advent of truth. In spirituality, it is believed that our thoughts and ideals shape our reality, and that we've have been given the power to show up our desires thru centered goal. Quantum physics similarly shows that the observer performs a crucial feature inside the appearance of fact, and that the act of looking a particle can exchange its conduct. This concept that we're co-creators of our fact is a effective one, and it indicates that we've extra manage over our lives than we'd apprehend.

The parallels amongst spirituality and quantum physics are fascinating and propose that there is a deeper level of fact past what we can see with our eyes. The thoughts of interconnectedness, the whole lot being strength, and the position of the observer in the arrival of truth are powerful requirements which have the ability to convert our statistics of ourselves and the universe.

Positive Affirmations... and BEYOND.

Positive affirmations are statements which you repeat to yourself to inspire incredible thinking and a super mind-set. They can be used to boost vanity, boom self notion, reduce pressure and anxiety, and reap non-public dreams. The power of first-rate affirmations lies within the truth that they allow you to reprogram your subconscious thoughts, which in turn can effect your mind, emotions, and behaviors. This isn't some element like the ones humans telling you to region up imaginative and prescient forums and all of your desires will come actual. What we are talking approximately right here is actual personal development this is sustainable and has the electricity to create a few thing you dream of. Every notable invention commenced as an concept, reputation creates ALL subjects.

To use powerful affirmations, begin via manner of the use of identifying the regions of your lifestyles that you want to beautify or change. Then, create affirmations which might be quality, unique, and plausible. For instance, as opposed to saying "I will in no way benefit achievement," say "I am a success and I will keep to benefit my desires."

Next, repeat your affirmations to yourself often, ideally inside the the front of a reflect. This will help you internalize the amazing messages and cause them to part of your unconscious mind. You also can write your affirmations down and location them in regions wherein you will see them frequently, together with on your rest room replicate or for your desk at artwork.

It's critical to phrase that pleasant affirmations by myself might not bring about trade to your life. You want to perform that and make terrific modifications in your conduct and conduct as nicely. However, extraordinary affirmations can be a effective device to help you live inspired and targeted on your desires, and to domesticate a extra super and optimistic mind-set.

Your mind is in reality an wonderful natural computer and whilst you jam it up with negativity at the same time as it comes time on the manner to achieve success, self sabotage hits you rectangular within the face. You want to every day remind yourself of everything exceptional approximately yourself, you don't stay in denial so you recognize wherein you need to make upgrades and you clearly modify.

In quit, superb affirmations are a smooth yet effective manner to enhance your thoughts-set and gain your goals. By repeating first-rate messages to your self regularly, you could reprogram your unconscious thoughts and domesticate a more best and powerful outlook on lifestyles. If you time table every day affirmations you are essentially programming the laptop that is your mind with codes for achievement.

Self-esteem is built through esteemable acts, self appreciate and self love are crucial on the equal time as constructing the a fulfillment person you're destined to be. Self-esteem is an essential factor of our highbrow fitness and properly-being. It refers to how we experience approximately ourselves, our skills, and our truely truely worth as humans. Having a healthy shallowness can assist us revel in more assured, capable, and resilient inside the face of existence's demanding situations. Here are a few pointers on a way to assemble shallowness.

Identify and assignment horrible ideals: Negative beliefs approximately ourselves may be deeply ingrained and frequently flow unchecked. Identify horrible self-communicate and undertaking it with evidence to the contrary.

Celebrate your accomplishments: Take time to reflect in your achievements, regardless of how small they will seem. Celebrating your successes builds self-self perception.

Practice self-care: Taking care of yourself bodily and mentally is important for building arrogance. Exercise frequently, devour healthily, and get enough relaxation.

Surround yourself with positivity: Surround your self with folks who deliver you up, and spend time in sports activities that bring you joy and achievement.

Set practicable dreams: Setting goals and walking within the direction of them can assist construct arrogance. Start small and constructing as lots as large goals.

Practice self-compassion: Treat yourself with kindness and information. Acknowledge that everyone makes mistakes and that failure is a natural a part of growth.

Building self-esteem is a manner that takes time and effort. But thru operating toward self-care, hard terrible beliefs, putting capacity goals, and surrounding yourself with positivity, you could cultivate a healthful and resilient sense of self confidence.

Chapter 16: Locating Yourself

I determined about this faculty course on happiness. The entire semester have turn out to be just on what humans said on their deathbeds that made them maximum satisfied in life and what they need they had completed greater of. The course came down to 2 subjects that made human beings maximum happy, one became doing selfless paintings. Doing topics for others, not for what you could get out of it, however actually to be of issuer to someone else. The 2nd, and I believe most crucial detail, changed into being your maximum real self. What the research had determined became that human beings being who they definitely are, no matter societal stressors to act in sure strategies, had been without a doubt satisfied.

The Importance of Being Yourself

Being yourself is one of the maximum essential subjects you could do in your intellectual fitness and well-being. When you're proper to yourself, you're more likely to feel assured, satisfied, and fulfilled. Here are a few motives why it's so important to be your self:

Authenticity: When you're authentic to your self, you are real. Authenticity approach that you are sincere, proper, and true to your values and ideals. People who're right are more likely to assemble robust relationships, have excessive vanity, and sense a feel of motive and which means in life.

Self-Acceptance: Being your self manner accepting who you are, flaws and all. When you take delivery of your self, you are more likely to be type to yourself, exercising self-compassion, and address your intellectual and physical fitness.

Confidence: When you're actual to yourself, you are much more likely to feel confident in your abilities and alternatives. This self assure assist you to navigate life's annoying conditions with resilience and perseverance. Do now not allow this section pass you via manner of, specifically in case you are a younger individual on the lookout for a reference to that particular every body. Confidence is one of the maximum important aspects to the early dating approach. If you are actually assured, and not surely sporting that fake bravado that most younger guys have, you will be a success in finding relationships, if you aren't a entire tool in a few special region.

Creativity: Being yourself method expressing your specific thoughts and perspectives. This creativity can purpose innovation, trouble-fixing, and private increase.

Happiness: When you are actual to your self, you are much more likely to pursue sports and relationships that deliver you pleasure and fulfillment. This happiness can result in a greater outstanding outlook on lifestyles and advanced highbrow fitness.

Tips for Being Yourself:

Identify your values and beliefs and stay with the useful resource of them.

Practice self-care and prioritize your intellectual and physical health.

Surround yourself with positivity and people who help and encourage you.

Embrace your strengths and weaknesses and get hold of them without judgment.

Pursue activities and relationships that align together collectively together with your actual self.

In stop, being yourself is vital for intellectual fitness, happiness, and private increase. It takes time and effort to construct self-interest and authenticity, however the blessings are definitely really worth it. Remember to be type to your self and have a good time your specific functions and views.

Now that you are assured, and characteristic a excellent revel in of self, how do I assemble actual self love and apprehend? Learning to like yourself is one of the maximum essential steps you may take in the direction of a happier and extra fascinating lifestyles. When you adore your self, you are more confident, resilient, and capable of face life's disturbing situations with grace and simplicity. However, it is not generally easy to love your self, specifically in case you've been through hard tales or struggle with self-doubt.

One of the primary steps towards studying to love yourself is to workout self-care. This approach searching after your physical, emotional, and highbrow fitness via using technique of getting enough sleep, consuming properly, exercising regularly, and taking time to do subjects that make you satisfied. When you prioritize your private dreams and properly-being, you're sending a message to yourself that you are valuable and deserving of love and care.

Another essential step is to find out and undertaking horrific self-speak. This is the voice in your head that tells you that you're no longer unique sufficient, that you're a failure, or that you don't deserve love and happiness. By turning into aware about this voice and actively hard it with wonderful affirmations and self-talk, you could start to retrain your thoughts to suppose greater genuinely about your self.

It's additionally important to surround yourself with positivity. This approach spending time with individuals who uplift and aid you, and preserving off those who deliver you down or make you experience terrible about yourself. When you surround your self with positivity, you are more likely to be ok with yourself and your life.

Another key to reading to love yourself is to encompass your strengths and weaknesses. We all have matters we're right at and subjects we warfare with, and that is adequate. By accepting and embracing each your strengths and weaknesses, you can discover ways to respect and love yourself for who you're, rather than continuously evaluating your self to others.

Finally, it's miles important to pursue sports and relationships that align along with your real self. This technique doing matters that make you happy and fulfilled, in desire to certainly doing what you believe you studied you "want to" be doing. By dwelling in alignment together in conjunction with your values and ideals, you may cultivate a feel of reason and which means that on your existence, which could contribute to greater self-love and happiness.

Learning to like your self is a adventure, and it may not appear in a single day. But with the aid of practicing self-care, difficult horrible self-speak, surrounding your self with positivity, embracing your strengths and weaknesses, and pursuing sports activities and relationships that align together with your real self, you could start to cultivate a deeper enjoy of self-love and attractiveness.

There are many procedures to head about finding yourself; there's meditation, excursion, training and our next problem count quantity: Mindfulness

Mindfulness is the exercise of being present, completely engaged, and aware about one's mind, emotions, and surroundings. It's the capability to have a study one's recollections without judgment, and it's far an essential tool for cultivating intellectual and emotional properly-being. In contemporary years, mindfulness has received reputation as a way for reducing stress, anxiety, and melancholy. Research has shown that working towards mindfulness can enhance intellectual fitness and bodily fitness, enhance cognitive characteristic, and sell emotional law.

One of the primary blessings of mindfulness is its capability to lessen stress. When we practice mindfulness, we attention our interest at the prevailing 2nd, which helps us to permit bypass of issues approximately the future or regrets approximately the past. This can decrease tiers of the stress hormone cortisol, which is associated with diverse terrible fitness outcomes, which encompass weight benefit, high blood stress, and immune tool disorder.

Another advantage of mindfulness is advanced emotional regulation. By becoming more privy to our mind and feelings, we're able to learn how to reply to them in a extra optimistic manner. This can assist us to control difficult feelings like anger, unhappiness, and tension, and save you them from overwhelming us. Mindfulness also can beautify our cognitive feature. When we exercise mindfulness, we train our brains to awareness our interest and clear out distractions. This can beautify reminiscence, mastering, and hassle-solving abilities.

In addition to the ones benefits, mindfulness can also sell feelings of properly-being and happiness. By learning to be gift and completely engaged in the present second, we will understand the easy pleasures of lifestyles and domesticate a enjoy of gratitude and contentment.

So how can we exercising mindfulness? There are many techniques, but a few commonplace ones encompass meditation, deep respiration wearing sports, and body reputation practices. These practices may be completed anywhere, at any time, and require no particular device or schooling.

Ultimately, mindfulness is a effective tool for non-public growth and emotional nicely-being. By cultivating interest and popularity of our experiences, we are capable of lessen pressure, improve emotional law, beautify cognitive characteristic, and sell happiness and nicely-being.

Building a Foundation of Self-Respect and Empathy

Self-recognize and empathy are fundamental dispositions that assist humans amplify wholesome and pleasant relationships with themselves and others. By constructing a sturdy basis of self-recognize and empathy, humans can enjoy a greater enjoy of self-worth, self-self perception, and emotional resilience. Self-admire consists of accepting and valuing oneself as a totally specific and valuable individual. It method treating oneself with kindness, compassion, and recognize, and refusing to accept a few thing a lot less than what one merits. Self-respect moreover consists of placing wholesome obstacles and status up for oneself while vital. Without self-apprehend, people may warfare with low self-esteem, self-doubt, and a lack of direction and reason in life.

Empathy, however, consists of data and sharing the emotions of others. It method being able to positioned oneself in a person else's shoes and relate to their evaluations and feelings. Empathy allows humans gather deeper connections with others, decorate communique and struggle decision talents, and boom a extra sense of compassion and kindness in the direction of others.

Building a basis of self-appreciate and empathy requires intentional try and exercising. Here are some tips for cultivating the ones inclinations:

Practice self-care: Self-care involves searching after one's physical, emotional, and intellectual well-being. This can embody getting enough sleep, ingesting a healthful food regimen, exercise frequently, and engaging in sports that deliver satisfaction and achievement.

Set boundaries: Setting boundaries way know-how one's limits and talking them to others. It method announcing "no" while a few element does now not revel in right, and status up for oneself on the identical time as vital.

Practice self-compassion: Self-compassion includes treating oneself with kindness and records, particularly within the direction of hard times. It technique recognizing that everyone makes errors and that it's miles k to ask for assist at the same time as wanted.

Practice energetic listening: Active listening includes paying complete hobby to what others are saying and validating their feelings and reviews. It technique heading off judgment and grievance and specializing in statistics and empathizing with others.

Practice gratitude: Gratitude involves appreciating the easy pleasures of life and recognizing the great in oneself and others. It method specializing in what one has in choice to what one lacks and cultivating a revel in of contentment and fulfillment.

By constructing a foundation of self-recognize and empathy, people can broaden a greater revel in of self-worth, emotional resilience, and healthful relationships with others. These tendencies require intentional attempt and exercise, however the blessings are properly properly virtually well worth it.

Self-actualization is the manner of information one's entire capability and conducting a revel in of achievement in life. It is the pinnacle of Maslow's Hierarchy of

Needs, which incorporates fundamental physiological needs, safety desires, love and belonging needs, and esteem desires. Self-actualization is the first-rate diploma of need, that could simplest be finished as speedy as all the other desires are met.

To achieve self-actualization, it's miles essential to be actual to oneself, pick out one's strengths and weaknesses, and set viable goals. Being proper to oneself requires a deep expertise of 1's values, beliefs, and goals. This way taking time to mirror on one's lifestyles, research, and relationships. It is also vital to apprehend and feature an first-rate time successes, no matter how small they'll seem.

Identifying strengths and weaknesses is important in the device of self-actualization. This manner being honest about one's capabilities and obstacles. It is critical to cognizance on strengths and use them to gather dreams, on the equal time as also strolling on weaknesses to decorate one's fundamental universal overall performance.

Setting capability goals is a few different important detail of self-actualization. Goals have to be specific, measurable, conceivable, relevant, and time-certain. This manner putting sensible goals which can be inner reap and align with one's values and ideals. Achieving those dreams will offer a experience of feat and satisfaction, that is essential for self-actualization.

Practicing self-compassion is also important within the way of self-actualization. This way treating oneself with kindness, know-how, and forgiveness. It is critical to be slight with yourself at the same time as going via demanding conditions or setbacks. Practicing self-compassion can assist to lessen pressure, tension, and depression, which can keep away from the approach of self-actualization.

Active listening is every other vital issue of self-actualization. This method listening to others with an open thoughts and without judgment. It is important to be absolutely gift and engaged in conversations, that could enhance relationships and foster a experience of empathy and records.

Gratitude is also essential in the machine of self-actualization. This way being grateful for what one has and appreciating the clean subjects in existence. Practicing gratitude can help to lessen stress, decorate temper, and foster a feel of nicely-being and contentment.

Self-actualization is the gadget of knowledge one's complete capability and mission a experience of success in life. It calls for being proper to one, figuring out strengths and weaknesses, setting capability desires, education self-compassion, lively listening, and gratitude. By incorporating the ones practices into one's lifestyles, people can enhance their emotional well-being, cognitive feature, and relationships with others.

Chapter 17: The Collective Conscious

As I channel my inner Fox Mulder I realize that the truth is available... But how do I find it? This subsequent thing goes to require a little suspension of disbelief, as we excursion into the paranormal. I might not have any peer reviewed studies to return up the findings of what is coming next however what I can can help you recognize is... while you pay attention the reality... you remember it.

The Akashic Records: A Gateway to Self-Discovery and Spiritual Growth

The Akashic Records are a metaphysical concept which has been known as the "Book of Life" or the "Universal Library." According to believers, the information encompass the statistics of every soul and its journey through time and vicinity. Accessing the Akashic Records is thought to provide a pathway to self-discovery, non secular growth, and statistics of the soul's reason.

The concept of the Akashic Records is rooted in ancient spiritual traditions, inclusive of

Hinduism, Buddhism, and Theosophy. The phrase "Akasha" is derived from the Sanskrit language and way "ether" or "area." The records are believed to exist in a higher size, beyond the bodily realm, and are accessed through meditation or different religious practices.

Accessing the Akashic Records calls for a deep degree of non secular cognizance and connection. It is said that each soul has a totally unique vibrational frequency this is used to get entry to the records. Some human beings get proper of entry to the data thru meditation or visualization, at the same time as others use techniques like automated writing or channeling.

There had been geniuses and prodigies which have stated their expertise have become truly divined to them with the resource of god himself. These highbrow behemoths should say they truely noticed the solutions seem in their minds as despite the fact that bestowed upon them like a gift from the most excessive.

The Akashic Records are believed to contain data approximately beyond lives, present occasions, and future possibilities. They are stated to embody data approximately soul contracts, karmic money owed, and spiritual lessons. Accessing the statistics can offer insight into one's purpose, relationships, and preferred life direction. Unfortunately, there has been no income succesful to expose us the manner to tap into those facts, I don't count on any of those lucky sufficient to have visible any part of the records have any concept how they have been linked. It seems to be a random present uncommon blessed people are given.

One of the benefits of having access to the Akashic Records is the opportunity for recuperation and personal increase. By data past lives and karmic styles, humans can release awful emotions and ideals that may be blockading their non secular evolution. The information also can offer steerage on a manner to flow forward in lifestyles and make choices that align with one's soul's motive.

It is important to observe that having access to the Akashic Records requires purpose and appreciate. It is not a exercising to be taken lightly, and it's miles essential to method it with humility and an open coronary coronary coronary heart. It is likewise vital to paintings with an authorized practitioner or instructor who can guide you through the approach and make sure that you are having access to the statistics accurately and ethically.

The Akashic Records are a effective tool for self-discovery and spiritual increase. They offer a gateway to know-how the soul's adventure and cause, further to an opportunity for recuperation and personal evolution. Accessing the facts calls for a deep degree of religious connection and goal, and it's far vital to approach the exercise with appreciate and steerage from an authorized practitioner. I wager when we enhance our abilities to each make use of our connection through quantum entanglement and faucet into the Akashic Records we will begin to see our complete capability. We have an extended manner to head however the human brain is an super organic laptop that we have simplest all commenced to apprehend.

To be able to attain excessive degrees of mental and religious acuity, one should be unmoved thru manner of life's troubles. I recognise that is a long way much less tough said than finished but it's far an important mission despite the truth that. When you are harassed out your frame releases the Cortisol enzyme, Cortisol reasons irritation, and contamination is the precursor to all illnesses. In brief, if you do not address strain and it over runs your lifestyles you may make your self bodily unwell. It is a reality that your highbrow usa may want to make you sick, however it can moreover heal you as properly. The placebo effect suggests you that the thoughts can heal you.

Stress Reduction

Stress is an unavoidable a part of existence; but, prolonged stress could have adverse consequences on our bodily, emotional, and highbrow fitness. The everyday barrage of stressors can bring about tension, despair, sleep troubles, or even continual illnesses like hypertension and diabetes. Therefore, it's miles important to understand the effect of pressure and feature a look at effective techniques to reduce it.

The Impact of Stress:

When we stumble upon a annoying state of affairs, our frame releases cortisol, a hormone that prepares the body for "combat or flight" reaction. In small doses, cortisol is essential for survival; however, continual stress can motive an overproduction of cortisol, that can wreak havoc on our frame. It can cause infection, weaken the immune system, and boom the danger of coronary heart disease, stroke, and different continual illnesses. Additionally, strain can effect our relationships, paintings productiveness, and normal top notch of existence.

How to Reduce Stress:

Fortunately, there are numerous effective processes to reduce pressure and sell common well-being. Here are a few realistic guidelines:

Practice Mindfulness: Once another time Mindfulness is the workout of being present in the second, without judgment. It can help us turn out to be more privy to our mind, feelings, and bodily sensations, and decrease the effect of pressure. Simple mindfulness practices like deep respiration, meditation, and yoga may be highly effective in reducing stress.

Exercise Regularly: Exercise is a high-quality pressure-buster. It releases endorphins, the feel-wonderful hormones, and reduces cortisol stages. It additionally lets in enhance sleep first-rate, this is important for strain good buy. Choose any physical hobby that you revel in, like dancing, swimming, or running, and make it part of your every day ordinary.

Get Enough Sleep: Lack of sleep can exacerbate stress and make it hard to deal with each day stressors. Make sure you get as a minimum 7-8 hours of uninterrupted sleep every night time time. Create a relaxing bedtime recurring, keep away from caffeine and electronics in advance than bedtime, and maintain your mattress room cool, dark, and quiet.

Connect with Loved Ones: Social help may be a effective pressure-reducer. Spend time with family and pals, interact in full-size conversations, and percentage your feelings and studies. It permit you to gain perspective, experience tested, and reduce feelings of isolation and loneliness. This is so critical and regularly ignored, your guide company is your tether to the relaxation of the area whilst you need area.

Practice Self-Care: Self-care is critical for pressure reduce price. Take day adventure for your self, interact in sports activities sports which you revel in, like analyzing, painting, or cooking. Take a heat bath, slight candles, or take note of soothing music. Nourish your frame with healthful, nutritious meals, and hydrate your self with hundreds of water.

In forestall, pressure is an inevitable part of lifestyles, however it's miles vital to govern it successfully to sell regular properly-being. Simple lifestyle adjustments like mindfulness practices, everyday workout, suitable sufficient sleep, social resource, and self-care can move an prolonged manner in lowering strain ranges. By prioritizing your intellectual and physical health, you can lead a happier, more wholesome, and further first-rate lifestyles.

As you learn how to lessen stress and anxiety you can locate that an prepared existence allows to unclutter your mental kingdom.

www.ingramcontent.com/pod-product-compliance
Lightning Source LLC
Chambersburg PA
CBHW070734020526
44118CB00035B/1346
* 9 7 8 0 9 9 5 8 6 1 0 5 3 *